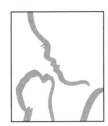

Acknowledgments

NRP Steering Committee Members
David Boyle, MD, FAAP, Co-chair, 2001–2005
Jeffrey M. Perlman, MB, ChB, FAAP, Co-chair, 2004–2006
Jay P. Goldsmith, MD, FAAP, Co-chair, 2005–2006
Marilyn Escobedo, MD, FAAP
Louis P. Halamek, MD, FAAP
George A. Little, MD, FAAP
Jane E. McGowan, MD, FAAP
Gary M. Weiner, MD, FAAP
Thomas E. Wiswell, MD, FAAP

Liaison Representatives
Jose Luis Gonzalez, MD, FACOG
    American College of Obstetricians and Gynecologists
Barbara Nightengale, RNC, NNP
    National Association of Neonatal Nurses
William A. Engle, MD, FAAP
    AAP Committee on Fetus and Newborn
Nalini Singhal, MD, FRCPC
    Heart and Stroke Foundation of Canada
Tim Myers, RRT-NPS
    American Association for Respiratory Care

The committee would like to express thanks to the following reviewers and contributors to this textbook:
American Academy of Pediatrics Committee on Fetus and Newborn
International Liaison Committee on Resuscitation, Neonatal Delegation
    Jeffrey M. Perlman, MB, ChB, FAAP, Co-chair
    Sam Richmond, MD, Co-chair
William Keenan, MD, FAAP, AAP Board-appointed Reviewer

American Heart Association Emergency Cardiovascular Care Leadership
Leon Chameides, MD, FAAP
Robert Hickey, MD, FAAP
Vinay Nadkarni, MD, FAAP
Mary Fran Hazinski, RN, MSN

American Heart Association Emergency Cardiovascular Care Pediatric Subcommittee
Arno Zaritsky, MD, FAAP, Chair, 2005–2006
Stephen M. Schexnayder, MD, FAAP, FCCM, Chair, 2003–2005
Dianne Atkins, MD, FAAP, FAHA
Robert Berg, MD, FAAP
Allan de Caen, MD, FRCPC
Ashrav Coovadia, MD
Douglas Diekema, MD, MPH, FAAP

American Heart Association Emergency Cardiovascular Care Pediatric Subcommittee *(continued)*
Michael J. Gerardi, MD, FAAP, FACEP
Monica Kleinman, MD, FAAP
Lester T. Proctor, MD, FAAP
Ricardo A. Samson, MD, FAAP
Anthony Scalzo, MD, FAAP
L. R. Tres Scherer III, MD, FAAP, FACS
Elise W. van der Jagt, MD, MPH, FAAP
Colleen Halverson, RN, MS

The Media Lab at Doernbecher Children's Hospital
Dana A. V. Braner, MD, FAAP
Ken Tegtmeyer, MD, FAAP
Susanna Lai, MPH
Richard Hodo

AAP Life Support Staff
Wendy Marie Simon, MA, CAE
Sheila Lazier, MEd
Kimberly Liotus
Bonnie Molnar
Kristy Goddyn
Tina Patel
Eileen Schoen

AAP Marketing and Publications Staff
Theresa Wiener
Sandi King

Copyeditor
Jill Rubino

NRP Education Workgroup Chair
Gary M. Weiner, MD, FAAP

Associated Education Materials for the *Textbook of Neonatal Resuscitation, 5th Edition*
Cases in Neonatal Resuscitation: Translating Knowledge and Skill Into Performance (video on DVD), Susan Niermeyer, MD, FAAP; Jeanette Zaichkin, RNC, MN; Gary M. Weiner, MD, FAAP; and Nalini Singhal, MD, FRCPC; Editors
Instructor's Manual for Neonatal Resuscitation, Jeanette Zaichkin, RNC, MN, Editor
NRP Slide Presentation Kit, Jay P. Goldsmith, MD, FAAP, Editor
NRP Written Evaluation Packet, Thomas E. Wiswell, MD, FAAP, and Jerry Short, PhD, Editors
NRP Reference Chart, Code Cart Cards, and Pocket Cards, Marilyn Escobedo, MD, FAAP, Editor

Contents

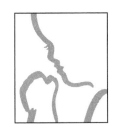

Preface

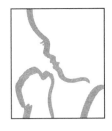

Birth is beautiful, miraculous, and probably the single most dangerous event that most of us will ever encounter in our lifetimes. Our bodies are required to make more radical physiologic adjustments immediately following birth than they will ever have to do again. It is remarkable that more than 90% of babies make the transition from intrauterine to extrauterine life perfectly smoothly, with little to no assistance required. It is for the remaining few percent that the Neonatal Resuscitation Program (NRP) was designed. While the percentage of newborns requiring assistance may be small, the real number of babies requiring help is substantial because of the large number of births. The implications of not receiving that help can be associated with problems that last a lifetime or even with death. The most gratifying aspect of providing skillful assistance to a compromised newborn is that your efforts are most likely to be successful, in contrast to the discouraging statistics associated with resuscitation attempts of adults or older children. The time that you devote to learning how to resuscitate newborns is time very well spent.

This textbook has a long history, with many pioneers from both the American Academy of Pediatrics (AAP) and the American Heart Association (AHA) responsible for its evolution. National guidelines for resuscitation of adults were initially recommended in 1966 by the National Academy of Sciences. In 1978, a Working Group on Pediatric Resuscitation was formed by the AHA Emergency Cardiac Care Committee. The group quickly concluded that resuscitation of newborns required a different emphasis than resuscitation of adults, with a focus on ventilation rather than cardiac defibrillation being paramount. The formal specialty of neonatology was evolving about that time and, by 1985, the AAP and the AHA expressed a joint commitment to develop a training program aimed at teaching the principles of neonatal resuscitation. The pioneering leaders of this effort were George Peckham and Leon Chameides. A committee was convened to determine the appropriate format for the program, and the material written by Ron Bloom and Cathy Cropley was selected to serve as the model for the new NRP textbook.

Pediatric leaders, such as Bill Keenan, Errol Alden, Ron Bloom, and John Raye, developed a strategy for disseminating the NRP. The strategy first involved training a national faculty consisting of at least one physician-nurse team from each state. The national faculty taught regional trainers who then trained hospital-based instructors. By the end of 2005, nearly 2 million health care providers in the United States had been trained in the techniques of neonatal resuscitation. The NRP also has been used as a model for similar neonatal resuscitation programs in 92 other countries.

The science behind the program has also undergone significant evolution. While the ABCD (Airway, Breathing, Circulation, Drugs) principles of resuscitation have been standard for several decades, the details of how and when to accomplish each of the steps and what to do differently for newborns versus older children or adults have required constant evaluation and change. Also, while the recommendations traditionally have been based on opinions from experts in the field, recently there has been a concerted effort to base the recommendations on experimental or experiential evidence, collected from studies performed in the laboratory, randomized control studies conducted in hospitals, and observational series systematically collected from clinicians.

The AHA has addressed this evaluation process by facilitating periodic international Cardiopulmonary Resuscitation and Emergency Cardiac Care (CPR-ECC) conferences every 5 to 8 years to establish guidelines for resuscitation of all age groups and for all causes of cardiopulmonary arrest. The AAP formally joined that process in 1992 for development of the guidelines for resuscitation of children and newborns.

The most recent CPR-ECC activity took place for more than 3 years and was conducted in 2 parts. First, starting in late 2002, a series of questions identifying controversial issues regarding resuscitation were identified by the International Liaison Committee on Resuscitation (ILCOR). Individual ILCOR members were then assigned to develop worksheets for each question. Advances in computerized databases and search engines facilitated the literature review and permitted the AHA to collect a detailed database of more than 30,000 references of publications regarding resuscitation. The

worksheets were debated in a series of conferences, following which a document entitled International Consensus on Cardiopulmonary Resuscitation (CPR) and Emergency Cardiovascular Care (ECC) Science With Treatment Recommendations (CoSTR) was published (*Circulation.* 2005;112:III-91–III-99). Second, each resuscitation council that makes up ILCOR was charged with developing resuscitation guidelines appropriate for the health care resources existing in its own region of the World, but based on the scientific principles defined in CoSTR. The neonatal portion of the US Treatment Guidelines was published in *Circulation, Resuscitation,* and *Pediatrics,* and is reprinted in the back of this textbook. As a result of this process, each successive edition of NRP contains more recommendations that are based on evidence, rather than simply reflecting common practice. We encourage you to review the evidence and, more importantly, to conduct the future studies necessary to further define the optimum practices.

The current edition of NRP has expanded content in several important areas, in response to comments collected from instructors and previous participants. It is well recognized that babies born prematurely

require assistance more often at birth and also present unique challenges to avoid complications that can have lifelong implications. In past editions, these challenges were addressed throughout the program, while now they have been collected in a separate lesson (Lesson 8). We also have listened to those who expressed concern that previous editions may have implied that all resuscitations should and will be successful, while the reality is that some babies born extremely early or with certain malformations are going to die despite the availability of optimum expertise. Therefore, another new lesson (Lesson 9) has been added to address ethical considerations and caring for infants, and families of babies who die. There also have been changes and reorganization within several of the first 7 lessons. A new Apgar Score recording form has been added to Lesson 1, Lesson 3 has been reorganized to place the details of the 2 types of resuscitation bags and the newer T-piece resuscitator into appendices, and a detailed description of the laryngeal mask airway has been added as an appendix for Lesson 5. Probably the most major change in content has been the approach to the use of supplemental oxygen. While the NRP continues to recommend using 100% oxygen whenever positive-pressure ventilation is required, the emphasis on always using high oxygen concentrations has been diminished and the use of oximeters and oxygen blenders for resuscitating very premature babies is recommended in the new Lesson 8. A change in the recommendation for epinephrine may also cause some confusion for those who were students of earlier editions. Previous editions taught that epinephrine can most easily be given via an endotracheal tube. However, recent research has shown that epinephrine is unpredictably absorbed from the lungs and may result in ineffective drug levels. One study suggested that as much as 10 times the intravenous dose may be required endotracheally to achieve the same serum level as could be achieved intravenously. Therefore, the current edition recommends the intravenous route as the preferred route, with endotracheal epinephrine given only while intravenous access is being established. Clinicians will need to be very careful not to confuse the new endotracheal dosing recommendations when administering the drug intravenously. There are other changes scattered throughout the program, so we encourage even the veteran students to read the entire new program.

Production of the NRP was accomplished through the efforts of a large number of people and several organizations. The collaborative relationships of the AHA, AAP, ILCOR, and the Pediatric Subcommittee of the AHA provided the infrastructure for developing recommendations that are more evidence-based and, therefore, internationally endorsed. The members of the NRP Steering Committee, listed in the front of this book, tirelessly debated the evidence and managed to reach consensus on a multitude of recommendations, while remaining sensitive to the practical implications of change. In particular, Gary Weiner is recognized for his description of the laryngeal mask airway and for drafting the foundation of the new Lesson 9. Bill Engle suggested a reorganization of Lesson 3 and added a new description of the T-piece resuscitator. Jane McGowan and Jeanette Zaichkin are superb pre-editors, with Jeanette constantly reminding us how the recommendations will be interpreted in the real world. Jill Rubino is thanked for her steadfast copyediting, Theresa Wiener for her production expertise, and Barbara Siede for her new drawings, many of which had to be reconstructed after their loss in the horrendous flood of New Orleans. While this textbook served as the content foundation, production of the supporting materials was accomplished only through the expertise and hard work of Lou Halamek (DVD and case filming), Susan Niermeyer (video), Ken Tegtmeyer and Dana Braner (DVD), Jeanette Zaichkin (instructor's manual, video, and slides), Jay Goldsmith (slides), Nalini Singhal (Megacode validation study), and Tom Wiswell (evaluations). Jerry Short has provided educational design expertise throughout the entire program. The leadership provided by Co-chairs David Boyle, Jeffrey Perlman, and Jay Goldsmith was excellent, with Jeff, in particular, being familiar with nearly every paper ever published on any element of neonatal resuscitation. I also want to thank Sam Richmond from the United Kingdom, who often went beyond his ILCOR obligations to suggest an international perspective to many aspects of the NRP presentation. Most importantly, everyone involved with the production of this complex and ambitious project will agree that one person is responsible for making each component fall into place and within the necessary time frame. Thank you, Wendy Simon, for all that you have done and continue to do.

John Kattwinkel, MD, FAAP

Neonatal Resuscitation Program Provider Course Overview

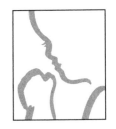

Neonatal Resuscitation Scientific Guidelines

The Neonatal Resuscitation Program (NRP) materials are based on the American Academy of Pediatrics (AAP) and American Heart Association (AHA) Guidelines for Cardiopulmonary Resuscitation and Cardiovascular Care of the Neonate (*Circulation*. 2005;112(suppl):IV-188–IV-195). The Guidelines were based on the International Liaison Committee on Resuscitation (ILCOR) consensus on science statement that was originally published in November 2005. A reprint of the Guidelines appears in the Appendix. Please refer to these pages if you have questions about the rationale for the current program recommendations. The evidence-based worksheets, prepared by members of ILCOR, which serve as the basis for both documents, can be viewed in the science area of the NRP Web site at www.aap.org/nrp.

Level of Responsibility

The standard-length NRP Provider Course consists of 9 lessons; however, you will need to work through only those lessons appropriate to your level of responsibility. Resuscitation responsibilities vary from hospital to hospital. For example, in some institutions, nurses may be responsible for intubating the newborn, but, in others, the physician or respiratory therapist may do so. The number of lessons you will need to complete depends on your personal level of responsibility.

Before starting the course, you must have a clear idea of your exact responsibilities. If you have any questions about the level of your responsibilities during resuscitation, please consult your instructor or supervisor.

Special Note: Neonatal resuscitation is most effective when performed by a designated and coordinated team. It is important for you to know the neonatal resuscitation responsibilities of team members who are working with you. Periodic practice among team members will facilitate coordinated and effective care of the newborn.

Lesson Completion

Successful completion of each lesson requires a passing score on the written evaluation for that lesson as well as successful completion of the Performance Checklist (for Lessons 2 through 6) and the Megacode. Upon successful completion of at least Lessons 1 through 4 <u>and</u> Lesson 9, participants are eligible to receive a Course Completion Card. This verification of participation is not issued on the day of the course. Instructors will distribute Course Completion Cards after the Course Roster is received and processed by the AAP Life Support staff.

Course participants may choose to use online testing (for a fee) to complete the written evaluation portion of the course. *However, participants must identify an instructor willing to provide performance evaluation **prior** to taking the online evaluation.* To learn more about online testing, please visit the NRP Web site at www.aap.org/nrp.

Completion Does Not Imply Competence

The Neonatal Resuscitation Program is an educational program that introduces the concepts and basic skills of neonatal resuscitation. Completion of the program does not imply that an individual has the competence to perform neonatal resuscitation. Each hospital is responsible for determining the level of competence and qualifications required for someone to assume clinical responsibility for neonatal resuscitation.

Standard Precautions

The US Centers for Disease Control and Prevention has recommended that standard precautions be taken whenever risk of exposure to blood or bodily fluids is high and the potential infectious status of the patient is unknown, as is certainly the case in neonatal resuscitation.

All fluid products from patients (blood, urine, stool, saliva, vomitus, etc) should be treated as potentially infectious. Gloves should be worn when resuscitating a newborn, and the rescuer should not use his or her mouth to apply suction via a suction device. Mouth-to-mouth resuscitation should be avoided by having a resuscitation bag and mask or a T-piece resuscitator always available for use during resuscitation. Masks and protective eyewear or face shields should be worn during procedures that are likely to generate droplets of blood or other bodily fluids. Gowns and aprons should be worn during procedures that will probably generate splashes of blood or other bodily fluids. Delivery rooms must be equipped with resuscitation bags, masks, laryngoscopes, endotracheal tubes, mechanical suction devices, and the necessary protective shields.

Textbook of Neonatal Resuscitation, 5th Edition, Interactive Multimedia DVD-ROM

The *Textbook of Neonatal Resuscitation, 5th Edition, Interactive Multimedia DVD-ROM* is located within this textbook. System requirements and content specifications are located on the inside front cover. In addition to all of the content and illustrations contained in the textbook, the DVD-ROM contains dramatic footage of actual resuscitation events, laryngoscopic view of the airway, digitized animation, and several multilevel, learner-directed, interactive video scenarios.

It is up to you to choose whether to learn the NRP content through reading the textbook, viewing the DVD-ROM, or a combination of the 2. However, the NRP Steering Committee highly encourages learners to make use of all resources available to them. The DVD-ROM offers great learning value, as it shows real-time video footage of the NRP steps and the learner-directed scenarios foster cognitive integration.

Overview and Principles of Resuscitation

The Neonatal Resuscitation Program (NRP) will help you learn to resuscitate newborns. By studying this book and practicing the skills, you will learn to be a valuable member of the resuscitation team.

Many concepts and skills are taught in the program. However, the single most important concept of the NRP emphasized throughout the program is that:

! **Ventilation of the baby's lungs is the most important and effective action in neonatal resuscitation.**

In Lesson 1 you will learn the

- **Changes in physiology that occur when a baby is born**

- **Sequence of steps to follow during resuscitation**

- **Risk factors that can help predict which babies will require resuscitation**

- **Equipment and personnel needed to resuscitate a newborn**

Why learn neonatal resuscitation?

Birth asphyxia accounts for about 19% of the approximately 5 million neonatal deaths that occur each year worldwide (World Health Organization, 1995). For many of these newborns, appropriate resuscitation was unavailable. Therefore, the outcomes of thousands of newborns per year might be improved by more widespread use of the resuscitation techniques taught in this program.

Which babies require resuscitation?

Approximately 10% of newborns require some assistance to begin breathing at birth; about 1% need extensive resuscitative measures to survive. In contrast, at least 90% of newly born babies make the transition from intrauterine to extrauterine life without difficulty. They require little to no assistance initiating spontaneous and regular respirations and completing the transition from the fetal to the neonatal blood-flow pattern.

ABCs of resuscitation
Airway (position and clear)
Breathing (stimulate to breathe)
Circulation (assess heart rate and color)

The "ABCs" of resuscitation are the same for babies as for adults. Ensure that the **A**irway is open and clear. Be sure that there is **B**reathing, whether spontaneous or assisted. Make certain that there is adequate **C**irculation of oxygenated blood. Newly born babies are wet following birth and heat loss is great. Therefore, it also is important to maintain body temperature during resuscitation.

The diagram below illustrates the relationship between resuscitation procedures and the number of newly born babies who need them. At the top are the procedures needed by all newborns. At the bottom are procedures needed by very few.

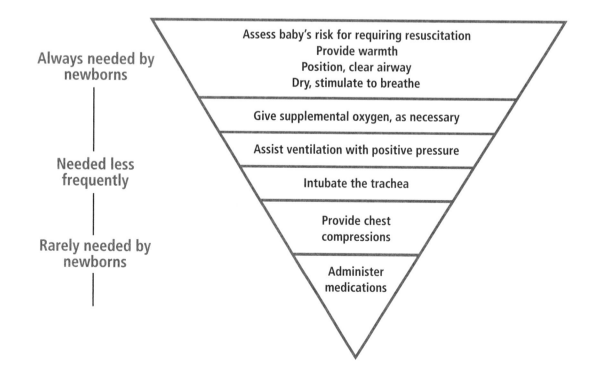

Always needed by newborns

Assess baby's risk for requiring resuscitation
Provide warmth
Position, clear airway
Dry, stimulate to breathe

Needed less frequently

Give supplemental oxygen, as necessary

Assist ventilation with positive pressure

Intubate the trachea

Rarely needed by newborns

Provide chest compressions

Administer medications

Every birth should be attended by someone who has been trained in initiating a neonatal resuscitation. Additional trained personnel will be necessary if a full resuscitation is required.

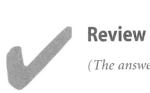

Review

(The answers are in the preceding section and at the end of the lesson.)

1. About _____% of newborns will require some assistance to begin regular breathing.

2. About _____% of newborns will require extensive resuscitation to survive.

3. Chest compressions and medications are (rarely) (frequently) needed when resuscitating newborns.

The Neonatal Resuscitation Program is organized in the following way:

Lesson 1: Overview and Principles of Resuscitation

Lesson 2: Initial Steps in Resuscitation

Lesson 3: Use of Resuscitation Devices for Positive-Pressure Ventilation

Lesson 4: Chest Compressions

Lesson 5: Endotracheal Intubation

Lesson 6: Medications

Lesson 7: Special Considerations

Lesson 8: Resuscitation of Babies Born Preterm

Lesson 9: Ethics and Care at the End of Life

You will have many opportunities to practice the steps involved in resuscitation and use the appropriate resuscitation equipment. You will gradually build your proficiency and speed. In addition, you will learn to evaluate a newborn throughout resuscitation and make decisions about what actions to take next.

In the next section, you will learn the basic physiology involved in a baby's transition from intrauterine to extrauterine life. Understanding the physiology of breathing and circulation in the newborn will help you understand why prompt resuscitation is vital.

How does a baby receive oxygen before birth?

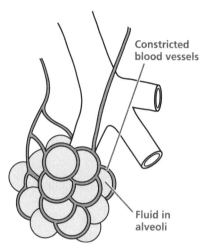

Figure 1.1. Fluid-filled alveoli and constricted blood vessels in the lung before birth

Oxygen is essential for survival both before and after birth. Before birth, all of the oxygen used by a fetus diffuses across the placental membrane from the mother's blood to the baby's blood.

Only a small fraction of fetal blood passes through the fetal lungs. The fetal lungs do not function as a source of oxygen or as a route to excrete carbon dioxide. Therefore, blood flow to the lungs is not important to maintain normal fetal oxygenation and acid-base balance. The fetal lungs are expanded in utero, but the potential air sacs (alveoli) within the lungs are filled with fluid, rather than air. In addition, the arterioles that perfuse the fetal lungs are markedly constricted, partly due to the low partial pressure of oxygen (pO_2) in the fetus (Figure 1.1).

Before birth, most of the blood from the right side of the heart cannot enter the lungs because of the increased resistance to flow in the constricted blood vessels in the fetal lungs. Instead, most of this blood takes the lower resistance path through the ductus arteriosus into the aorta (Figure 1.2).

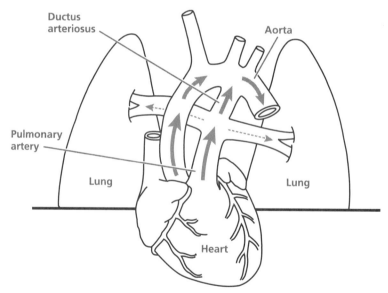

Figure 1.2. Shunting of blood through the ductus arteriosus and away from the lungs before birth

After birth, the newborn will no longer be connected to the placenta and will depend on the lungs as the only source of oxygen. Therefore, in a matter of seconds, the lung fluid must be absorbed from the alveoli, the lungs must fill with air that contains oxygen, and the blood vessels in the lungs must relax to increase blood flow to the alveoli so that oxygen can be absorbed and carried to the rest of the body.

What normally happens at birth to allow a baby to get oxygen from the lungs?

Normally, 3 major changes begin immediately after birth.

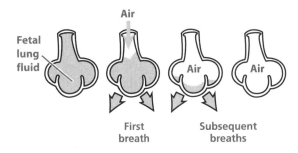

1. The **fluid in the alveoli is absorbed** into lung tissue and replaced by air (Figure 1.3). Because air contains 21% oxygen, filling the alveoli with air provides oxygen that can diffuse into the blood vessels that surround the alveoli.

Figure 1.3. Fluid replaced by air in alveoli

2. The **umbilical arteries and vein constrict and then are clamped.** This removes the low-resistance placental circuit and increases systemic blood pressure.

3. As a result of the gaseous distention and increased oxygen in the alveoli, the **blood vessels in the lung tissue relax, decreasing resistance to blood flow** (Figure 1.4). This relaxation, together with the increased systemic blood pressure, results in a lower pressure in the pulmonary

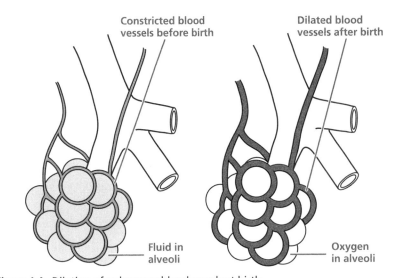

Figure 1.4. Dilation of pulmonary blood vessels at birth

arteries than in the systemic circulation and leads to a dramatic increase in pulmonary blood flow and a decrease in flow through the ductus arteriosus. The oxygen from the alveoli is absorbed by the blood in the pulmonary vessels, and the oxygen-enriched blood returns to the left side of the heart, where it is pumped to the tissues of the newborn's body.

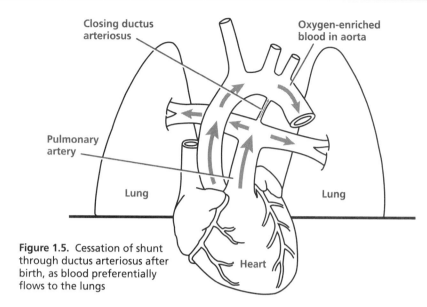

Figure 1.5. Cessation of shunt through ductus arteriosus after birth, as blood preferentially flows to the lungs

In most circumstances, air provides sufficient oxygen (21%) to initiate relaxation of the pulmonary blood vessels. As blood levels of oxygen increase and pulmonary blood vessels relax, the ductus arteriosus begins to constrict. Blood previously diverted through the ductus arteriosus now flows through the lungs, where it picks up more oxygen to transport to tissues throughout the body (Figure 1.5).

At the completion of this normal transition, the baby is breathing air and using his lungs to get oxygen. His initial cries and deep breaths have been strong enough to help move the fluid from his airways. The oxygen and gaseous distention of the lungs are the main stimuli for the pulmonary blood vessels to relax. As adequate oxygen enters the blood, the baby's skin turns from gray/blue to pink.

Although the initial steps in a normal transition occur within a few minutes of birth, the entire process may not be completed until hours or even several days after delivery. For example, studies have shown that, in normal transition of term newborns, it may take up to 10 minutes to achieve an oxygen saturation of 90% or greater. Complete closure of the ductus arteriosus may not occur until 12 to 24 hours after birth, and complete relaxation of the lung vessels does not occur for several months.

What can go wrong during transition?

A baby may encounter difficulty before labor, during labor, or after birth. If the difficulty begins in utero, either before or during labor, the problem usually reflects compromise in the uterine or placental blood flow. The first clinical sign can be a deceleration of the fetal heart rate, which may return to normal even after blood flow has been significantly compromised. Problems encountered after birth are more likely to involve the baby's airway and/or lungs. The following are some of the problems that may disrupt normal transition:

- The baby may not breathe sufficiently to force fluid from the alveoli, or material such as meconium may block air from entering the alveoli. As a result, the lungs may not fill with air, preventing oxygen from reaching the blood circulating through the lungs (hypoxemia).

- Excessive blood loss may occur, or there may be poor cardiac contractility or bradycardia from hypoxia and ischemia, so that the expected increase in blood pressure cannot occur (systemic hypotension).

- A failure of gaseous distention of the lungs or lack of oxygen may result in sustained constriction of the pulmonary arterioles, thus decreasing the blood flow to the lungs and oxygen supply to body tissues. In some cases, the pulmonary arterioles may fail to relax even after the lungs are filled with air/oxygen (persistent pulmonary hypertension of the newborn, frequently abbreviated as PPHN).

How does a baby respond to an interruption in normal transition?

Normally, the newborn makes vigorous efforts to inhale air into the lungs. The pressure created assists fetal lung fluid to move out of the alveoli and into the surrounding lung tissue. This also brings oxygen to the pulmonary arterioles and causes the arterioles to relax. If this sequence is interrupted, the pulmonary arterioles can remain constricted, the alveoli remain filled with fluid instead of air, and the systemic arterial blood may not become oxygenated.

When oxygen supply is decreased, the arterioles in the bowels, kidneys, muscles, and skin constrict, while blood flow to the heart and brain remains stable or increases to maintain oxygen delivery. This redistribution of blood flow helps preserve function of the vital organs. However, if oxygen deprivation continues, myocardial function and cardiac output deteriorate, blood pressure falls, and blood flow to all organs is reduced. The consequence of this lack of adequate blood perfusion and tissue oxygenation can be irreversible brain damage, damage to other organs, or death.

The compromised baby may exhibit 1 or more of the following clinical findings:

- Poor muscle tone from insufficient oxygen delivery to the brain, muscles, and other organs
- Depression of respiratory drive from insufficient oxygen delivery to the brain
- Bradycardia (slow heart rate) from insufficient delivery of oxygen to the heart muscle or brain stem
- Low blood pressure from insufficient oxygen to the heart muscle, blood loss, or insufficient blood return from the placenta before or during birth
- Tachypnea (rapid respirations) from failure to absorb fetal lung fluid
- Cyanosis (blue color) from insufficient oxygen in the blood

Many of these same symptoms also may occur in other conditions, such as infection or hypoglycemia, or if the baby's respiratory efforts have been depressed by medications, such as narcotics or general anesthetic agents, given to the mother before birth.

How can you tell if a newborn had in utero or perinatal compromise?

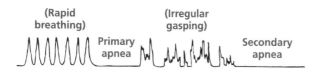

Figure 1.6. Primary and secondary apnea

Laboratory studies have shown that cessation of respiratory efforts is the first sign that a newborn is deprived of oxygen. After an initial period of rapid breathing attempts, a period of *primary apnea* occurs (Figure 1.6), during which stimulation, such as drying or slapping the newborn's feet, will cause a resumption of breathing.

However, if oxygen deprivation continues during primary apnea, the baby will make several attempts to gasp and then will enter a period of *secondary apnea* (Figure 1.6). During secondary apnea, stimulation will *not* restart the baby's breathing. Assisted ventilation must be provided to reverse the process triggered by oxygen deprivation.

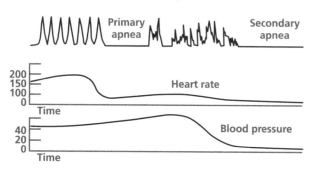

Heart rate begins to fall at about the same time that the baby enters primary apnea. Blood pressure is usually maintained until the onset of secondary apnea (unless blood loss has resulted in an earlier onset of hypotension) (Figure 1.7).

Figure 1.7. Heart rate and blood pressure changes during apnea

 If a baby does not begin breathing immediately after being stimulated, he or she is likely in secondary apnea and will require positive-pressure ventilation. Continued stimulation will not help.

Most of the time, the baby will be presented to you somewhere in the middle of the sequence described above. Often, the compromising event will have started before or during labor. Therefore, at the time of birth, it will be difficult to determine how long the baby has been compromised. Physical examination will not allow you to distinguish between primary and secondary apnea. However, the respiratory response to stimulation may help you estimate how recently the event began. If the baby begins breathing as soon as he is stimulated, he was in primary apnea; if he does not breathe right away, he is in secondary apnea. As a general rule, the longer a baby has been in secondary apnea, the longer it will take for spontaneous breathing to resume. However, the graph in Figure 1.8 demonstrates that, as soon as ventilation is established, most compromised newborns usually will show a very rapid improvement in heart rate.

If effective positive-pressure ventilation does not result in a rapid increase in heart rate, the duration of the compromising event may have been such that myocardial function has deteriorated and blood pressure has fallen below a critical level. Under these circumstances, chest compressions and, possibly, medications will be required for resuscitation.

Review

(The answers are in the preceding section and at the end of the lesson.)

4. Before birth, the alveoli in a baby's lungs are (collapsed) (expanded) and filled with (fluid) (air).

5. The air that fills the baby's alveoli during normal transition contains _____% oxygen.

6. The oxygen in the baby's lungs then causes the pulmonary arterioles to (relax) (constrict) so that the oxygen can be absorbed from the alveoli and distributed to all organs.

7. If a baby does not begin breathing in response to stimulation, you should assume he is in _____ apnea and you should provide _____.

8. If a baby is deprived of oxygen and he enters the stage of secondary apnea, his heart rate will (rise) (fall) and his blood pressure will (rise) (fall).

9. Restoration of adequate ventilation usually will result in a (rapid) (gradual) (slow) improvement in heart rate.

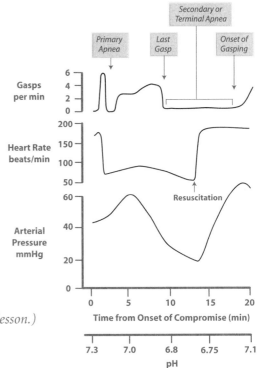

Figure 1.8. Sequence of physiological events in animal models from multiple species involving complete total asphyxia. Note the prompt increase in heart rate as soon as resuscitation is begun.

The resuscitation flow diagram

This flow diagram describes all of the NRP resuscitation procedures. The diagram begins with the birth of the baby. Each resuscitation step is shown in a block. Below each block is a decision point to help you decide if you need to proceed to the next step.

Study the diagram as you read the description of each step and decision point. This diagram will be repeated in later lessons. Use it to help you remember the steps involved in a resuscitation.

Initial Assessment Block. At the time of birth, you should ask yourself 4 questions about the newborn. These questions are shown in the Assessment block of the diagram. If any answer is "No," you should continue to the initial steps of resuscitation.

Ⓐ *Block A (Airway).* These are the initial steps you take to establish an **A**irway and begin resuscitating a newborn.

- Provide warmth.
- Position the head to open the airway; clear the airway as necessary.
- Dry the skin, stimulate the baby to breathe, and reposition the head to open the airway.

Note how quickly you evaluate the baby and take the initial steps. As the time line shows, you should complete these blocks in about 30 seconds.

Evaluation of the effect of Block A. You evaluate the newborn after about 30 seconds. You should simultaneously evaluate respirations, heart rate, and color. If the newborn is not breathing adequately (has apnea or is gasping), has a heart rate of less than 100 beats per minute (bpm), or appears blue (cyanotic), you proceed to 1 of the 2 Blocks B.

Ⓑ *Block B (Breathing).* If the baby has apnea or has a heart rate below 100 bpm, you assist the baby's **B**reathing by providing positive-pressure ventilation. If he is cyanotic, you may give him supplemental oxygen.

Evaluation of the effect of Block B. After about 30 seconds of ventilation and/or supplemental oxygen, you evaluate the newborn again. If the heart rate is below 60 bpm, you proceed to Block C.

Ⓒ *Block C (Circulation).* You support **C**irculation by starting chest compressions while continuing positive-pressure ventilation.

Evaluation of the effect of Block C. After about 30 seconds of chest compressions and positive-pressure ventilation, you evaluate the newborn again. If the heart rate is still below 60 bpm, you proceed to Block D.

Ⓓ *Block D (Drug).* You administer epinephrine as you continue positive-pressure ventilation and chest compressions.

Evaluation of Block D. If the heart rate remains below 60 bpm, the actions in Blocks C and D are continued and repeated. This is indicated by the curved arrow.

Be sure that each step is being performed correctly and effectively before proceeding to the next step.

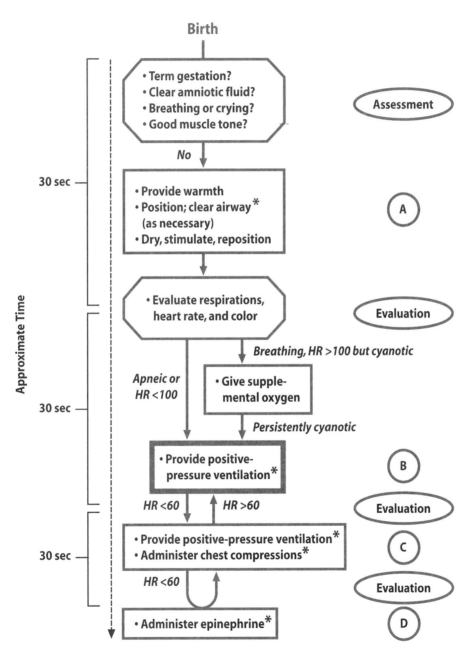

* Endotracheal intubation may be considered at several steps.

When the heart rate improves and rises above 60 bpm, chest compressions are stopped. Positive-pressure ventilation is continued until the heart rate is above 100 bpm and the baby is breathing.

Please note the following important points about the flow diagram:

- There are 2 heart rates to remember: 60 bpm and 100 bpm. In general, a heart rate below 60 bpm indicates that additional resuscitation steps are needed. A heart rate above 100 bpm usually indicates that resuscitation procedures beyond those in Block A can be stopped, unless the patient is apneic.

- The asterisks (*) in the flow diagram indicate points at which endotracheal intubation may be needed. These points will be described in later lessons.

- The time line beside the flow diagram indicates how quickly resuscitation proceeds from step to step. If you are sure resuscitation is being performed effectively, do not continue a step beyond about 30 seconds when a newborn shows no improvement. Instead, proceed to the next step in the flow diagram. If you feel that any step is not being delivered effectively, you may need to take longer than 30 seconds to correct the problem.

- The primary actions in neonatal resuscitation are aimed at ventilating the baby's lungs (Blocks A and B). Once this has been accomplished, heart rate, blood pressure, and pulmonary blood flow usually will improve spontaneously. However, if blood and tissue oxygen levels are low, cardiac output may have to be assisted by chest compressions and epinephrine (Blocks C and D) for blood to reach the lungs to pick up oxygen.

Now take time to become familiar with the flow diagram, and learn the order of steps that will be presented in the following lessons. Also learn the heart rates you use to decide if the next step is needed.

Look at the color photographs in the center of the book (Center Pages A through F). The newborn in Figure A-1 has all the characteristics of a vigorous baby born at term. The newborn in Figure B-2 has poor muscle tone and color and requires resuscitation.

How do you prioritize your actions?

Evaluation is based primarily on the following 3 signs:

- Respirations
- Heart rate
- Color

You will decide whether a particular step is effective by assessing each of these 3 signs. Although you will evaluate all 3 signs simultaneously, a seriously low heart rate is most important for determining whether you should proceed to the next step. This process of evaluation, decision, and action is repeated frequently throughout resuscitation.

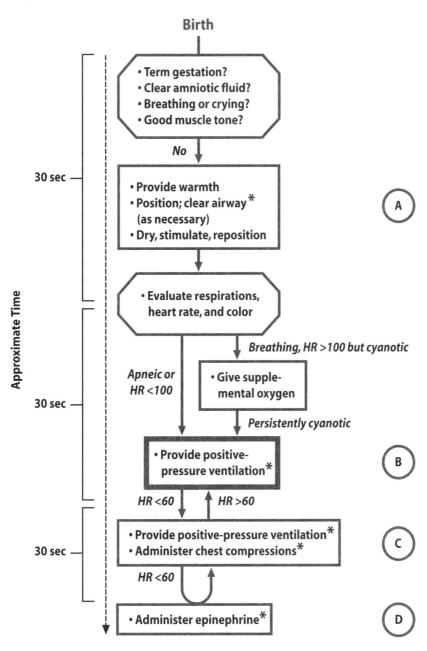

Birth

- Term gestation?
- Clear amniotic fluid?
- Breathing or crying?
- Good muscle tone?

No

30 sec

- Provide warmth
- Position; clear airway* (as necessary)
- Dry, stimulate, reposition

A

- Evaluate respirations, heart rate, and color

Breathing, HR >100 but cyanotic

Apneic or HR <100

- Give supplemental oxygen

30 sec

Persistently cyanotic

- Provide positive-pressure ventilation*

B

HR <60   *HR >60*

- Provide positive-pressure ventilation*
- Administer chest compressions*

C

30 sec

HR <60

- Administer epinephrine*

D

*Endotracheal intubation may be considered at several steps.

Approximate Time

* Endotracheal intubation may be considered at several steps.

Why is the Apgar score *not* used to guide resuscitation?

The Apgar score is an objective method of quantifying the newborn's condition and is useful for conveying information about the newborn's overall status and response to resuscitation. However, resuscitation must be initiated before the 1-minute score is assigned. Therefore, ***the Apgar score is not used to determine the need for resuscitation, what resuscitation steps are necessary, or when to use them.*** The 3 signs that you will use to decide how and when to resuscitate (respirations, heart rate, and color) do form part of the score. Two additional elements (muscle tone and reflex irritability) reflect neurologic status. It should be noted that the values of the individual elements of the score will be different if the baby is being resuscitated; therefore, the record should indicate what resuscitation measures, if any, are being taken each time the score is assigned.

The Apgar score normally is assigned at 1 minute and again at 5 minutes of age. When the 5-minute score is less than 7, additional scores should be assigned every 5 minutes for up to 20 minutes. Although the Apgar score is not a good predictor of outcome, the change of score at sequential time points following birth can reflect how well the baby is responding to resuscitative efforts. Elements of the Apgar score are described in the Appendix at the end of this lesson.

How do you prepare for a resuscitation?

At every birth, you should be prepared to resuscitate a newborn because the need for resuscitation can come as a complete surprise. For this reason, every birth should be attended by at least 1 person skilled in neonatal resuscitation whose only responsibility is management of the newborn. Additional personnel will be needed if more complex resuscitation is anticipated.

With careful consideration of risk factors, more than half of all newborns who will need resuscitation can be identified prior to birth. If you anticipate the possible need for neonatal resuscitation, you should

- Recruit additional skilled personnel to be present.
- Prepare the necessary equipment.

What risk factors are associated with the need for neonatal resuscitation?

Review this list of risk factors.
Consider having a copy readily available in the labor and delivery areas.

Antepartum Factors

Maternal diabetes
Pregnancy-induced hypertension
Chronic hypertension
Fetal anemia or isoimmunization
Previous fetal or neonatal death
Bleeding in second or third trimester
Maternal infection
Maternal cardiac, renal, pulmonary, thyroid, or neurologic disease
Polyhydramnios
Oligohydramnios
Premature rupture of membranes
Fetal hydrops

Post-term gestation
Multiple gestation
Size-dates discrepancy
Drug therapy, such as
    Magnesium
    Adrenergic-blocking drugs
Maternal substance abuse
Fetal malformation or anomalies
Diminished fetal activity
No prenatal care
Age <16 or >35 years

Intrapartum Factors

Emergency cesarean section
Forceps or vacuum-assisted delivery
Breech or other abnormal presentation
Premature labor
Precipitous labor
Chorioamnionitis
Prolonged rupture of membranes (>18 hours before delivery)
Prolonged labor (>24 hours)
Prolonged second stage of labor (>2 hours)
Macrosomia

Persistent fetal bradycardia
Non-reassuring fetal heart rate patterns
Use of general anesthesia
Uterine hyperstimulation
Narcotics administered to mother within 4 hours of delivery
Meconium-stained amniotic fluid
Prolapsed cord
Abruptio placentae
Placenta previa
Significant intrapartum bleeding

Why are premature babies at higher risk?

Many of these risk factors may result in a baby being born before 37 completed weeks of gestation. Premature babies have anatomical and physiological characteristics that are quite different from babies born at term. These characteristics include

- Lungs deficient in surfactant, which may make ventilation difficult
- Immature brain development, which may decrease the drive to breathe
- Weak muscles, which may make spontaneous breathing more difficult
- Thin skin, large surface area, and decreased fat, which all contribute to rapid heat loss
- Higher likelihood of being born with an infection
- Very fragile blood vessels in the brain, which may bleed during periods of stress
- Small blood volume, making them more susceptible to the hypovolemic effects of blood loss
- Immature tissues, which may be more easily damaged by excessive oxygen

These and other aspects of prematurity should alert you to seek extra help when anticipating a preterm birth. The details and precautions associated with resuscitation of a premature baby will be presented in Lesson 8.

What personnel should be present at delivery?

At every delivery, there should be at least 1 person who can be immediately available to the baby as his or her only responsibility and who is capable of initiating resuscitation. Either this person or someone else who is immediately available should have the skills required to perform a complete resuscitation, including endotracheal intubation and administration of medications. It is not sufficient to have someone "on call" (either at home or in a remote area of the hospital) for newborn resuscitations in the delivery room. When resuscitation is needed, it must be initiated without delay.

If the delivery is anticipated to be high risk, and thus may require more advanced neonatal resuscitation, at least 2 persons should be present solely to manage the baby—1 with complete resuscitation skills and 1 or more to assist. The concept of a "resuscitation team," with a specified leader and an identified role for each member, should be the goal. For multiple births, a separate team should be organized for each baby.

For example, if a delivery room nurse is present at an uncomplicated birth, this nurse might initially clear the airway, provide tactile stimulation, and evaluate the respirations and heart rate. If the newborn does not respond appropriately, the nurse would initiate positive-pressure ventilation and call for assistance. A second person would help assess the efficacy of positive-pressure ventilation. A physician or nurse with full resuscitation skills would be in the immediate vicinity and available to intubate the trachea and assist with coordinated chest compressions and ventilation, and to order medication.

In the case of an anticipated high-risk birth, 2, 3, or even 4 people with varying degrees of resuscitation skills may be needed at the delivery. One of them, with complete resuscitation skills, would serve as the leader of the team and would probably be the one to position the baby, open the airway, and intubate the trachea, if necessary. Two others would assist with positioning, suctioning, drying, and giving oxygen. They could administer positive-pressure ventilation or chest compressions as directed by the leader. A fourth person would be helpful for administering medications and/or documenting the events.

Remember that a birth is associated with blood and other body fluids, and a neonatal resuscitation provides considerable opportunity for transmission of infectious agents. Be sure that all personnel observe appropriate standard precautions as defined by hospital policy and Occupational Safety & Health Administration (OSHA) regulations.

What equipment should be available?

All the equipment necessary for a complete resuscitation must be in the delivery room and be fully operational. When a high-risk newborn is expected, appropriate equipment should be ready to use. A complete list of neonatal resuscitation equipment is in the Appendix at the end of this lesson.

What do you do after a resuscitation?

Babies who have required resuscitation are at risk for deterioration after their vital signs have returned to normal. You learned earlier in this lesson that the longer a baby has been compromised, the longer he or she will take to respond to resuscitation efforts. The NRP will refer to the following 3 levels of post-resuscitation care:

Routine Care: Nearly 90% of newborns are vigorous term babies with no risk factors and with clear amniotic fluid. They do not need to be separated from their mothers after birth to receive the equivalent of the initial steps of resuscitation. Thermoregulation can be provided by putting the baby directly on the mother's chest, drying, and covering with dry linen. Warmth is maintained by direct skin-to-skin contact with the mother. Clearing of the upper airway can be provided as necessary by wiping the baby's mouth and nose. While the initial steps can be provided in modified form, ongoing observation of breathing, activity, and color must be carried out to determine the need for additional intervention.

Observational Care: Babies who have prenatal or intrapartum risk factors, have meconium staining of the amniotic fluid or skin, have depressed breathing or activity, and/or are cyanotic will need closer assessment. These babies should be evaluated and managed initially under a radiant warmer and should receive the initial steps as appropriate. These babies are still at risk for developing problems associated with perinatal compromise and should be evaluated *frequently* during the immediate neonatal period. In many cases, this will involve admitting the baby to a transitional area of the newborn nursery where cardiorespiratory monitoring is available and vital signs may be taken frequently. However, parents should be permitted and encouraged to see, touch, and possibly hold their baby, depending on the degree of stability.

Post-resuscitation Care: Babies who require positive-pressure ventilation or more extensive resuscitation may require ongoing support, are at high risk for recurrent deterioration, and are at high risk for developing subsequent complications of an abnormal transition. These babies generally should be managed in an environment where ongoing evaluation and monitoring are available. Transfer to an intensive care nursery may be necessary. Parents also should be given liberal access to their baby in these settings. Details of post-resuscitation care will be presented in Lesson 7.

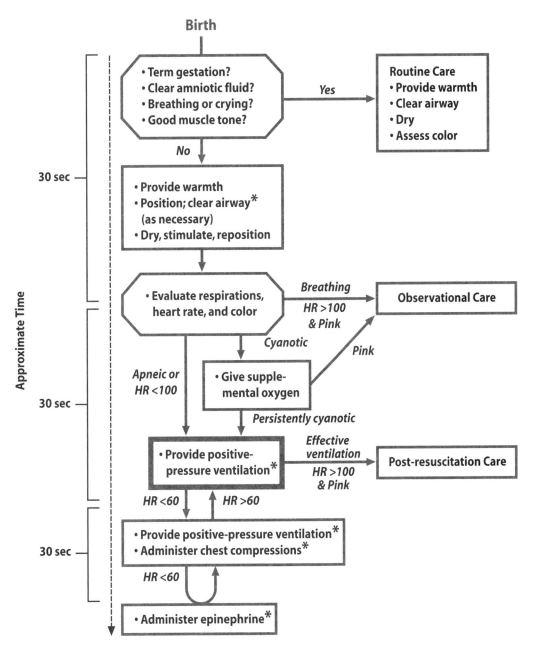

Birth

- Term gestation?
- Clear amniotic fluid?
- Breathing or crying?
- Good muscle tone?

Yes →

Routine Care
- Provide warmth
- Clear airway
- Dry
- Assess color

No

- Provide warmth
- Position; clear airway*
  (as necessary)
- Dry, stimulate, reposition

- Evaluate respirations,
  heart rate, and color

Breathing
HR >100 & Pink → **Observational Care**

Cyanotic

Apneic or HR <100

- Give supple-
  mental oxygen

Pink → **Observational Care**

Persistently cyanotic

- Provide positive-
  pressure ventilation*

Effective ventilation
HR >100 & Pink → **Post-resuscitation Care**

HR <60   *HR >60*

- Provide positive-pressure ventilation*
- Administer chest compressions*

HR <60

- Administer epinephrine*

Approximate Time

30 sec

30 sec

30 sec

* Endotracheal intubation may be considered at several steps.

Review

(The answers are in the preceding section and at the end of the lesson.)

10. Complete the missing parts of the chart.

    A. Apnea or heart rate < _____

    B. Provide _____

    C. Heart rate < _____

    D. Provide positive-pressure ventilation and _____

    _____

    E. Heart rate < _____

11. Resuscitation (should) (should not) be delayed until the 1-minute Apgar score is available.

12. Premature babies may present unique challenges during resuscitation because of
    A. Fragile brain capillaries that may bleed
    B. Lungs deficient in surfactant, making ventilation difficult
    C. Poor temperature control
    D. Higher likelihood of an infection
    E. All of the above

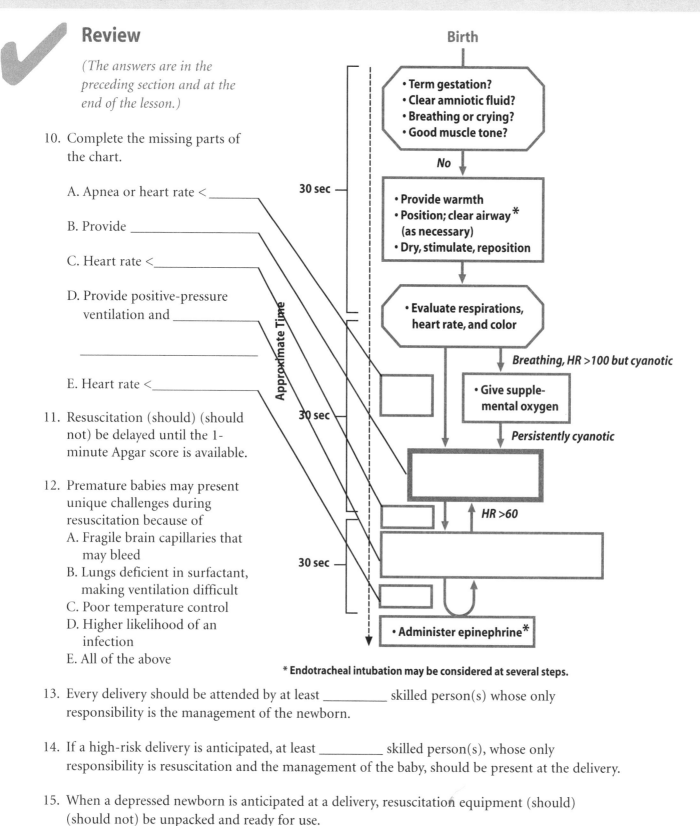

* Endotracheal intubation may be considered at several steps.

13. Every delivery should be attended by at least _____ skilled person(s) whose only responsibility is the management of the newborn.

14. If a high-risk delivery is anticipated, at least _____ skilled person(s), whose only responsibility is resuscitation and the management of the baby, should be present at the delivery.

15. When a depressed newborn is anticipated at a delivery, resuscitation equipment (should) (should not) be unpacked and ready for use.

16. A baby who was meconium stained and not vigorous at birth had meconium suctioned from the trachea. She then resumed breathing and became more active. This baby should now receive (routine) (observational) (post-resuscitation) care.

Key Points

1. Most newly born babies are vigorous. Only about 10% require some kind of assistance and only 1% need major resuscitative measures (intubation, chest compressions, and/or medications) to survive.

2. The most important and effective action in neonatal resuscitation is to ventilate the baby's lungs.

3. Lack of ventilation of the newborn's lungs results in sustained constriction of the pulmonary arterioles, preventing systemic arterial blood from becoming oxygenated. Prolonged lack of adequate perfusion and oxygenation to the baby's organs can lead to brain damage, damage to other organs, or death.

4. When a fetus/newborn first becomes deprived of oxygen, an initial period of attempted rapid breathing is followed by primary apnea and dropping heart rate that will improve with tactile stimulation. If oxygen deprivation continues, secondary apnea ensues, accompanied by a continued fall in heart rate and blood pressure. Secondary apnea cannot be reversed with stimulation; assisted ventilation must be provided.

5. Initiation of effective positive-pressure ventilation during secondary apnea usually results in a rapid improvement in heart rate.

6. The majority of, but not all, neonatal resuscitations can be anticipated by identifying the presence of antepartum and intrapartum risk factors associated with the need for neonatal resuscitation.

7. All newborns require initial assessment to determine whether resuscitation is required.

8. Every birth should be attended by at least 1 person whose only responsibility is the baby and who is capable of initiating resuscitation. Either that person or someone else who is immediately available should have the skills required to perform a complete resuscitation. When resuscitation is anticipated, additional personnel should be present in the delivery room before the delivery occurs.

9. Resuscitation should proceed rapidly.
   • You have approximately 30 seconds to achieve a response from one step before deciding whether you need to go on to the next.
   • Evaluation and decision making are based primarily on respirations, heart rate, and color.

Key Points — *continued*

10. The steps of neonatal resuscitation are as follows:

    A. Initial steps.
    - Provide warmth.
    - Position head and clear airway as necessary.*
    - Dry and stimulate the baby to breathe.
    - Evaluate respirations, heart rate, and color.

    B. Provide positive-pressure ventilation with a resuscitation bag and supplemental oxygen.*

    C. Provide chest compressions as you continue assisted ventilation.*

    D. Administer epinephrine as you continue assisted ventilation and chest compressions.*

    *Consider intubation of the trachea at these points.

Lesson 1 Review

(The answers follow.)

1. About _____% of newborns will require some assistance to begin regular breathing.

2. About _____% of newborns will require extensive resuscitation to survive.

3. Chest compressions and medications are (rarely) (frequently) needed when resuscitating newborns.

4. Before birth, the alveoli in a baby's lungs are (collapsed) (expanded) and filled with (fluid) (air).

5. The air that fills the baby's alveoli during normal transition contains _____% oxygen.

6. The oxygen in the baby's lungs then causes the pulmonary arterioles to (relax) (constrict) so that the oxygen can be absorbed from the alveoli and distributed to all organs.

7. If a baby does not begin breathing in response to stimulation, you should assume he is in _____ apnea and you should provide _____.

8. If a baby is deprived of oxygen and he enters the stage of secondary apnea, his heart rate will (rise) (fall), and his blood pressure will (rise) (fall).

9. Restoration of adequate ventilation usually will result in a (rapid) (gradual) (slow) improvement in heart rate.

Lesson 1 Review — *continued*

10. Complete the missing parts of the chart.

    A. Apnea or heart rate < _____

    B. Provide _____

    C. Heart rate < _____

    D. Provide positive-pressure ventilation and _____

    E. Heart rate < _____

11. Resuscitation (should) (should not) be delayed until the 1-minute Apgar score is available.

12. Premature babies may present unique challenges during resuscitation because of
    A. Fragile brain capillaries that may bleed
    B. Lungs deficient in surfactant, making ventilation difficult
    C. Poor temperature control
    D. Higher likelihood of an infection
    E. All of the above

13. Every delivery should be attended by at least _____ skilled person(s) whose only responsibility is the management of the newborn.

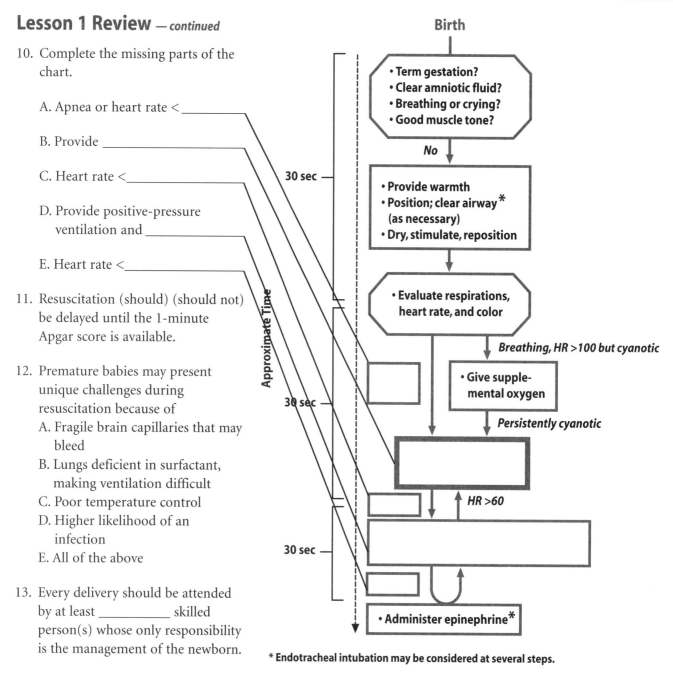

Birth

- **Term gestation?**
- **Clear amniotic fluid?**
- **Breathing or crying?**
- **Good muscle tone?**

No

- **Provide warmth**
- **Position; clear airway*** **(as necessary)**
- **Dry, stimulate, reposition**

- **Evaluate respirations, heart rate, and color**

Breathing, HR >100 but cyanotic

- **Give supplemental oxygen**

Persistently cyanotic

HR >60

- **Administer epinephrine***

Approximate Time

30 sec

30 sec

30 sec

* **Endotracheal intubation may be considered at several steps.**

14. If a high-risk delivery is anticipated, at least _____ skilled person(s), whose only responsibility is resuscitation and the management of the baby, should be present at the delivery.

15. When a depressed newborn is anticipated at a delivery, resuscitation equipment (should) (should not) be unpacked and ready for use.

16. A baby who was meconium stained and not vigorous at birth had meconium suctioned from the trachea. She then resumed breathing and became more active. This baby should now receive (routine) (observational) (post-resuscitation) care.

Lesson 1 Answers to Questions

1. 10%.

2. 1%.

3. Chest compressions and medications are **rarely** needed when resuscitating newborns.

4. Before birth, the alveoli are **expanded** and filled with **fluid.**

5. The air that fills the baby's alveoli during normal transition contains **21%** oxygen.

6. Oxygen causes pulmonary arterioles to **relax.**

7. You should assume **secondary apnea** and you should provide **positive-pressure ventilation.**

8. The baby's heart rate will **fall,** and his blood pressure will **fall.**

9. Ventilation usually will result in a **rapid** improvement in heart rate.

10. A. Apnea or Heart rate <**100 beats per minute.**
    B. Provide **positive-pressure ventilation.**
    C. Heart rate <**60 beats per minute.**
    D. Provide positive-pressure ventilation and **chest compressions.**
    E. Heart rate <**60 beats per minute.**

11. Resuscitation **should not** be delayed until the 1-minute Apgar score is available.

12. Premature babies have fragile brain capillaries, immature lungs, and poor temperature control, and are more likely to have an infection. Therefore, **all of the above** is the correct answer.

13. Every delivery should be attended by at least **1** skilled person.

14. At least **2** skilled persons should be present at a high-risk delivery.

15. Equipment **should** be unpacked if a newborn is anticipated to be depressed at delivery.

16. Since the baby required suctioning of meconium from the airway, she should receive **observational** care.

Appendix

Neonatal Resuscitation Supplies and Equipment

Suction equipment

Bulb syringe

Mechanical suction and tubing

Suction catheters, 5F or 6F, 8F, 10F, 12F or 14F

8F feeding tube and 20-mL syringe

Meconium aspirator

Bag-and-mask equipment

Device for delivering positive-pressure ventilation, capable of
delivering 90% to 100% oxygen

Face masks, newborn and premature sizes (cushioned-rim masks
preferred)

Oxygen source with flowmeter (flow rate up to 10 L/min) and
tubing

Intubation equipment

Laryngoscope with straight blades, No. 0 (preterm) and No. 1
(term)

Extra bulbs and batteries for laryngoscope

Endotracheal tubes, 2.5-, 3.0-, 3.5-, 4.0-mm internal diameter (ID)

Stylet (optional)

Scissors

Tape or securing device for endotracheal tube

Alcohol sponges

CO_2 detector or capnograph

Laryngeal mask airway (optional)

Medications

Epinephrine 1:10,000 (0.1 mg/mL) — 3-mL or 10-mL ampules

Isotonic crystalloid (normal saline or Ringer's lactate) for volume
expansion — 100 or 250 mL

Sodium bicarbonate 4.2% (5 mEq/10 mL) — 10-mL ampules

Naloxone hydrochloride 0.4 mg/mL — 1-mL ampules, or
1.0 mg/mL — 2-mL ampules

Dextrose 10%, 250 mL

Normal saline for flushes

Umbilical vessel catheterization supplies

    Sterile gloves

    Scalpel or scissors

    Antiseptic prep solution

    Umbilical tape

    Umbilical catheters, 3.5F, 5F

    Three-way stopcock

Syringes, 1, 3, 5, 10, 20, 50 mL

Needles, 25, 21, 18 gauge, or puncture device for needleless system

Neonatal Resuscitation Supplies and Equipment — *continued*

Miscellaneous

Gloves and appropriate personal protection

Radiant warmer or other heat source

Firm, padded resuscitation surface

Clock with second hand (timer optional)

Warmed linens

Stethoscope (neonatal head preferred)

Tape, 1/2 or 3/4 inch

Cardiac monitor and electrodes or pulse oximeter and probe (optional for delivery room)

Oropharyngeal airways (0, 00, and 000 sizes or 30-, 40-, and 50-mm lengths)

For very preterm babies (optional)

Compressed air source

Oxygen blender to mix oxygen and compressed air

Pulse oximeter and oximeter probe

Reclosable, food-grade plastic bag (1-gallon size) or plastic wrap

Chemically activated warming pad

Transport incubator to maintain baby's temperature during move to the nursery

Apgar Score

The Apgar score describes the condition of the newborn infant immediately after birth and, when properly applied, provides a standardized mechansim to record fetal-to-neonatal transition. Each of the 5 signs is awarded a value of 0, 1, or 2. The 5 values are then added and the sum becomes the Apgar score. Resuscitative interventions modify the components of the Apgar score; therefore, the resuscitative measures being administered at the time the score is assigned should also be registered. A suggested form for completion at deliveries is shown in the following table:

APGAR SCORE

Gestational Age _____ weeks

SIGN	0	1	2	1 minute	5 minutes	10 minutes	15 minutes	20 minutes
Color	Blue or Pale	Acrocyanotic	Completely Pink					
Heart Rate	Absent	<100 minute	>100 minute					
Reflex irritability	No Response	Grimace	Cry or Active Withdrawal					
Muscle Tone	Limp	Some Flexion	Active Motion					
Respiration	Absent	Weak Cry; Hypoventilation	Good, crying					
			TOTAL					

Comments:	Resuscitation					
	Minutes	1	5	10	15	20
	Oxygen					
	PPV/NCPAP					
	ETT					
	Chest Compressions					
	Epinephrine					

Apgar scores should be assigned at 1 minute and 5 minutes after birth. When the 5-minute score is less than 7, additional scores should be assigned every 5 minutes for up to 20 minutes. These scores should not be used to dictate appropriate resuscitative actions, nor should interventions for depressed infants be delayed until the 1-minute assessment. The scores should be recorded in the baby's birth record. Complete documentation of the events taking place during a resuscitation must also include a narrative description of interventions performed.

Initial Steps
in Resuscitation

In Lesson 2 you will learn how to

- Decide if a newborn needs to be resuscitated.
- Open the airway, and provide the initial steps of resuscitation.
- Resuscitate a newborn when meconium is present.
- Provide free-flow oxygen when needed.

The following 2 cases are examples of how the initial steps of evaluation and resuscitation may be used. As you read each case, imagine yourself as part of the resuscitation team. The details of the initial steps will be described in the remainder of the lesson.

Case 1.
An uncomplicated delivery

A 24-year-old woman enters the hospital in active labor at term. Membranes ruptured 1 hour before, and the amniotic fluid was clear. The cervix dilates progressively and, after several hours, a baby boy is born vaginally in vertex presentation.

The cord is clamped and cut. Clear secretions are cleaned from the baby's mouth and nose. He begins to cry as he is dried with a warm towel.

He quickly becomes pink, has good muscle tone, and is placed on his mother's chest to remain warm and to complete transition.

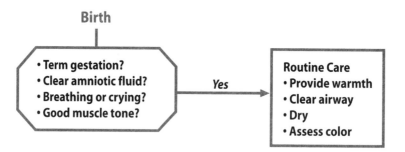

Case 2.
Resuscitation involving meconium

A multiparous woman presents at term in early labor. Soon after admission, her membranes rupture, and the fluid is noted to contain thick meconium, similar to "pea soup." Fetal heart rate monitoring shows occasional late decelerations. A judgment is made to allow a vaginal delivery.

After the baby is completely born, he has poor tone, minimal respiratory efforts, and central cyanosis. He is placed under a radiant warmer while his oropharynx is cleared of meconium with a large-bore suction catheter. The trachea is intubated and suction is applied to the endotracheal tube as it is being removed from the trachea, but no meconium is recovered. The baby still has weak respiratory efforts.

The baby is now dried with a warm towel and stimulated to breathe by flicking the soles of his feet. At the same time, his head is repositioned to establish his airway. He immediately begins to breathe more effectively, and the heart rate is measured to be more than 120 beats per minute (bpm). Because he is still cyanotic, he is given supplemental oxygen by holding an oxygen mask, providing 100% oxygen, close to his face.

By 10 minutes after birth, the baby is breathing regularly and the supplemental oxygen is gradually withdrawn. He now has a heart rate of 150 bpm, and remains pink without supplemental oxygen. Several minutes later, he is placed on his mother's chest to continue transition while vital signs and activity are observed closely and monitored frequently for possible deterioration.

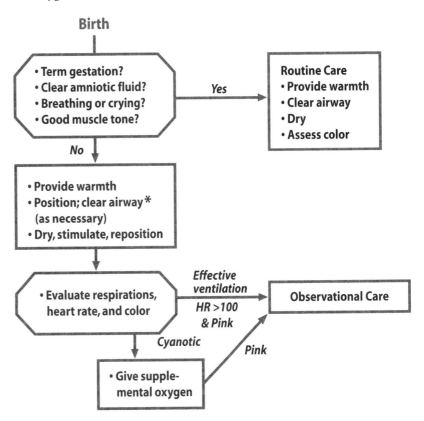

* Endotracheal intubation may be indicated at this point to clear meconium from the trachea.

How do you determine if a baby requires resuscitation?

* Term gestation?
* Clear amniotic fluid?
* Breathing or crying?
* Good muscle tone?

• *Was the baby born at term?*

Although more than 90% of babies will complete intrauterine to extrauterine transition without requiring any assistance, the vast majority of these babies will be born at term. If the baby was born preterm, there is a significantly higher likelihood that some degree of resuscitation will be required. For example, preterm babies are more likely to have stiff, underdeveloped lungs, may have insufficient muscle strength to make strong initial respiratory efforts, and have less capacity to maintain body temperature after birth. Therefore, preterm babies should be evaluated and offered the initial steps of resuscitation, separate from the mother and under a radiant warmer. If the baby is only slightly preterm and is judged to have stable vital signs, he can then be returned to his mother's chest within several minutes to complete transition. Details of management of the unstable preterm baby will be covered in Lesson 8.

• *Was the amniotic fluid clear?*

This is a very important question. The amniotic fluid should be clear, showing no signs of containing meconium. Babies who are very stressed in utero will often pass meconium into the amniotic fluid. If meconium is present and the baby is not vigorous, it will be necessary to intubate the trachea to clear it of meconium before the baby takes many breaths. If the amniotic fluid is clear, or if the meconium-stained baby is vigorous, suctioning the trachea will not be necessary. No more than a few seconds should elapse while you make this determination.

• *Is the baby breathing or crying?*

Breathing is evident by watching the baby's chest. A vigorous cry also indicates breathing. However, don't be misled by a baby who is gasping. Gasping is a series of deep single or stacked inspirations that occur in the presence of hypoxia and/or ischemia. It is indicative of severe neurologic and respiratory depression.

 Gasping usually indicates a significant problem and requires the same intervention as no respiratory efforts at all (apnea).

• *Is there good muscle tone?*

Healthy term babies should have flexed extremities and be active.

What are the initial steps and how are they administered?

If the baby is term and vigorous, the initial steps may be provided in modified form, as described in Lesson 1 (page 1-18 under "Routine Care").

Once you decide that resuscitation is required, all of the initial steps should be initiated within a few seconds. Although they are listed as "initial" and are given in a particular order, they should be applied throughout the resuscitation process.

• *Provide warmth*
The baby should be placed under a radiant warmer so that the resuscitation team has easy access to the baby and the radiant heat helps reduce heat loss (Figure 2.1). The baby should not be covered with blankets or towels. Leave the baby uncovered to allow full visualization and to permit the radiant heat to reach the baby.

• *Position by slightly extending the neck*
The baby should be **positioned** on the back or side, with the neck slightly extended in the "sniffing" position. This will bring the posterior pharynx, larynx, and trachea in line and facilitate unrestricted air entry. This alignment in the supine position is also the best position for assisted ventilation with a bag and mask and/or the placement of an endotracheal tube. The goal is to move the baby's nose as far anterior as possible, thus creating the "sniffing" position.

Care should be taken to prevent hyperextension or flexion of the neck, since either may restrict air entry (Figure 2.2).

> **Initial Steps**
> - Provide warmth
> - Position; clear airway (as necessary)
> - Dry, stimulate, reposition

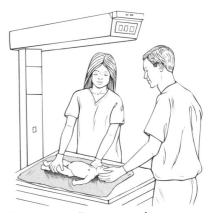

Figure 2.1. Radiant warmer for resuscitating newborns

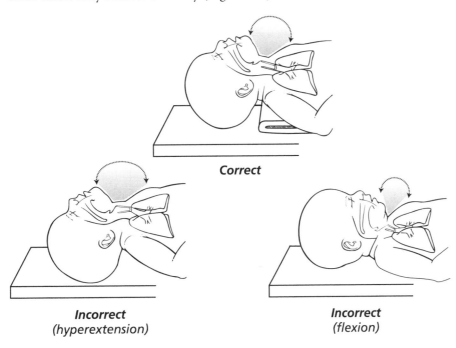

Correct

Incorrect
(hyperextension)

Incorrect
(flexion)

Figure 2.2. Correct and incorrect head positions for resuscitation

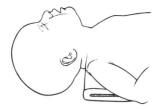

Figure 2.3. Optional shoulder roll for maintaining "sniffing" position

To help maintain the correct position, you may place a rolled blanket or towel under the shoulders (Figure 2.3). This shoulder roll may be particularly useful if the baby has a large occiput (back of head) resulting from molding, edema, or prematurity.

• *Clear airway (as necessary)*

After delivery, the appropriate method for clearing the airway further will depend on

1. The presence of meconium

2. The baby's level of activity

Study the flow diagram below to understand how you suction newborns who are meconium stained.

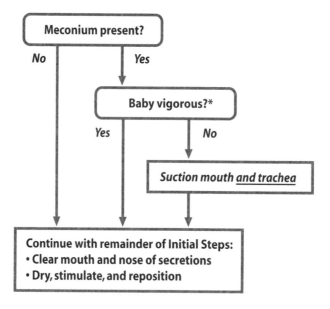

* Vigorous is defined as strong respiratory efforts, good muscle tone, and a heart rate greater than 100 bpm. The technique of determining the heart rate is described later in this lesson.

What do you do if meconium is present and the baby is *not* vigorous?

If the baby born with meconium-stained fluid has depressed respirations, depressed muscle tone, and/or a heart rate less than 100 bpm, direct suctioning of the trachea soon after delivery is indicated before many respirations have occurred. The following steps can reduce the chances of the baby developing meconium aspiration syndrome—a very serious respiratory disorder:

• Insert a laryngoscope and use a 12F or 14F suction catheter to clear the mouth and posterior pharynx so that you can visualize the glottis (Figure 2.4).

• Insert an endotracheal tube into the trachea.

- Attach the endotracheal tube to a suction source. (A special aspirator device will be needed.) (Figure 2.4)

- Apply suction as the tube is slowly withdrawn.

- Repeat as necessary until little additional meconium is recovered, or until the baby's heart rate indicates that resuscitation must proceed without delay.

Details of performing endotracheal intubation and suctioning are described in Lesson 5. Individuals who will be initiating resuscitation, but who will not be intubating newborns, should still be competent in assisting with endotracheal intubation. This also is described in Lesson 5.

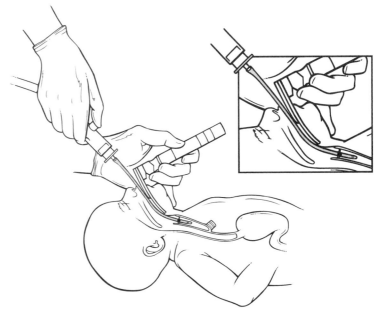

Figure 2.4. Visualizing the glottis and suctioning meconium from the trachea using a laryngoscope and endotracheal tube (see Lesson 5 for details)

Note: Some previous recommendations have suggested that endotracheal suctioning should be determined by whether the meconium has "thick," versus "thin," consistency. While it may be reasonable to speculate that thick meconium might be more hazardous than thin, there are currently no clinical studies that warrant basing suctioning guidelines on meconium consistency.

Also, various techniques, such as squeezing the chest, inserting a finger in the baby's mouth, or externally occluding the airway, have been proposed to prevent babies from aspirating meconium. None of these techniques have been subjected to rigorous research evaluation, and all may be harmful to the baby. They are not recommended.

What do you do if meconium is present and the baby *is* vigorous?

If the baby born with meconium-stained fluid has a normal respiratory effort, normal muscle tone, and a heart rate greater than 100 bpm, simply use a bulb syringe or large-bore suction catheter to clear secretions and any meconium from the mouth and nose. This procedure is described in the next section.

Review

(The answers are in the preceding section and at the end of the lesson.)

1. A newborn who is born at term, has no meconium in the amniotic fluid or on the skin, is breathing well, and has good muscle tone (does) (does not) need resuscitation.

2. A newborn with meconium in the amniotic fluid and who **is not vigorous** (will) (will not) need to have a laryngoscope inserted and be suctioned with an endotracheal tube. A newborn with meconium in the amniotic fluid and who **is vigorous** (will) (will not) need to have a laryngoscope inserted and be suctioned with an endotracheal tube.

3. When deciding which babies need tracheal suctioning, the term "vigorous" is defined by what 3 characteristics?

   (1)_____

   (2)_____

   (3)_____

4. When a suction catheter is used to clear the oropharynx of meconium before inserting an endotracheal tube, the appropriate size is _____F or _____F.

5. Which drawing shows the correct way to position a newborn's head prior to suctioning the airway?

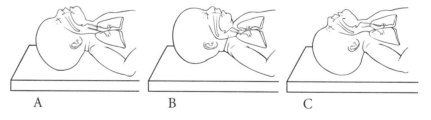

| A | B | C |

6. A newborn is covered with meconium, is breathing well, has normal muscle tone, has a heart rate of 120 beats per minute, and is pink. The correct action is to

   _____ Insert a laryngoscope and suction his trachea with an endotracheal tube.

   _____ Suction the mouth and nose with a bulb syringe or suction catheter.

How do you clear the airway if no meconium is present?

Secretions may be removed from the airway by wiping the nose and mouth with a towel or by suctioning with a bulb syringe or suction catheter. If the newborn has copious secretions coming from the mouth, turn the head to the side. This will allow secretions to collect in the cheek where they can more easily be removed.

Use a bulb syringe or a catheter attached to mechanical suction to remove fluid that appears to be blocking the airway. When using suction from the wall or from a pump, the suction pressure should be set so that, when the suction tubing is blocked, the negative pressure (vacuum) reads approximately 100 mm Hg.

The mouth is suctioned before the nose to ensure that there is nothing for the newborn to aspirate if he or she should gasp when the nose is suctioned. You can remember "mouth before nose" by thinking "M" comes before "N" in the alphabet (Figure 2.5). If material in the mouth and nose is not removed before the newborn breathes, the material can be aspirated into the trachea and lungs. When this occurs, the respiratory consequences can be serious.

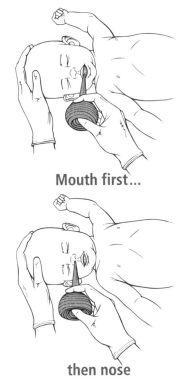

Mouth first...

then nose

Figure 2.5. Suctioning the mouth and nose; "M" before "N"

! **Caution: When you suction, particularly when using a catheter, be careful not to suction vigorously or deeply. Stimulation of the posterior pharynx during the first few minutes after birth can produce a vagal response, causing severe bradycardia or apnea. Brief, gentle suctioning with a bulb syringe usually is adequate to remove secretions.**

If bradycardia occurs during suctioning, stop suctioning and reevaluate the heart rate.

Suctioning, in addition to clearing the airway to allow unrestricted air entry to the lungs, also provides a degree of *stimulation*. In some cases, this is all the stimulation needed to initiate respirations in the newborn.

Once the airway is clear, what should be done to prevent further heat loss and to stimulate breathing?

• *Dry, stimulate to breathe, and reposition*

Often, positioning the baby and suctioning secretions will provide enough stimulation to initiate breathing. Drying will also provide stimulation. Drying the body and head will also help prevent heat loss. If 2 people are present, the second person can be drying the baby while the first person is positioning and clearing the airway.

As part of preparation for a resuscitation, you should have several pre-warmed absorbent towels or blankets available. The baby is initially placed on one of these towels, which can be used to dry most of the fluid. This towel should then be discarded, and fresh pre-warmed towels or blankets should be used for continued drying and stimulation.

While you dry the baby, and thereafter, be sure to keep the head in the "sniffing" position to maintain a good airway (Figure 2.6).

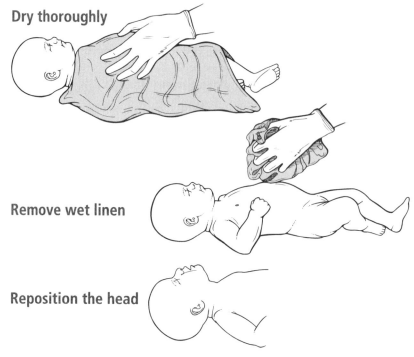

Dry thoroughly

Remove wet linen

Reposition the head

Figure 2.6. Drying and removing wet linen to prevent heat loss and repositioning the head to ensure an open airway

What other forms of stimulation may help a baby breathe?

Both drying and suctioning stimulate the newborn. For many newborns, these steps are enough to induce respirations. If the newborn does not have adequate respirations, additional tactile stimulation may be provided *briefly* to stimulate breathing.

It is important to understand the correct methods of tactile stimulation. Stimulation may be useful not only to encourage a baby to begin breathing during the initial steps of resuscitation, but also may be used to stimulate continued breathing after positive-pressure ventilation.

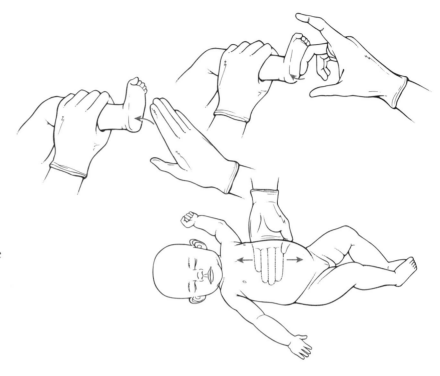

Figure 2.7. Acceptable methods of stimulating a baby to breathe

Safe and appropriate methods of providing additional tactile stimulation include

- Slapping or flicking the soles of the feet
- Gently rubbing the newborn's back, trunk, or extremities (Figure 2.7)

 Overly vigorous stimulation is not helpful and can cause serious injury. Do not shake the baby.

Remember, if a newborn is in primary apnea, almost any form of stimulation will initiate breathing. If a baby is in secondary apnea, no amount of stimulation will work. Therefore, 1 or 2 slaps or flicks to the soles of the feet, or rubbing the back once or twice, should be sufficient. If the newborn remains apneic, positive-pressure ventilation should be initiated immediately, as described in Lesson 3.

Continued use of tactile stimulation in a newborn who is not breathing wastes valuable time. For persistent apnea, give positive-pressure ventilation.

What forms of stimulation may be hazardous?

Certain actions that were used in the past to provide tactile stimulation to apneic newborns can harm a baby and should not be used.

Harmful Actions	Potential Consequences
Slapping the back or buttocks	Bruising
Squeezing the rib cage	Fractures, pneumothorax, respiratory distress, death
Forcing thighs onto abdomen	Rupture of liver or spleen
Dilating anal sphincter	Tearing of anal sphincter
Using hot or cold compresses or bath	Hyperthermia, hypothermia, burns
Shaking	Brain damage

Review

(The answers are in the preceding section and at the end of the lesson.)

7. In suctioning a baby's nose and mouth, the rule is to first suction the _____ and then the _____.

8. Make a check mark next to the correct ways to stimulate a newborn.

 _____ Slap on the back   _____ Slap on the sole of foot

 _____ Rub the back   _____ Squeeze the rib cage

9. If a baby is in secondary apnea, stimulation alone (will) (will not) stimulate breathing.

10. A newborn is still not breathing after a few seconds of stimulation. The next action should be to administer

 _____ Additional stimulation

 _____ Positive-pressure ventilation

Now that you have warmed, positioned, cleared the airway, dried, stimulated, and repositioned the baby's head, what do you do next?

Evaluate the baby

Your next step is to evaluate the newborn to determine if further resuscitation actions are indicated. The vital signs that you evaluate are as follows:

• *Respirations*

There should be good chest movement, and the rate and depth of respirations should increase after a few seconds of tactile stimulation.

 Remember, gasping respirations are ineffective and require the same intervention as for apnea.

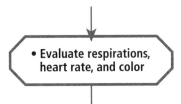
• Evaluate respirations, heart rate, and color

• *Heart rate*

The heart rate should be more than 100 bpm. The easiest and quickest method to determine the heart rate is to feel for a pulse at the base of the umbilical cord, where it attaches to the baby's abdomen (Figure 2.8). However, sometimes the umbilical vessels are constricted so that the pulse is not palpable. Therefore, if you cannot feel a pulse, you should listen for the heartbeat over the left side of the chest using a stethoscope. If you can feel a pulse or hear the heartbeat, tap it out on the bed so that others will also know the heart rate.

Counting the number of beats in 6 seconds and multiplying by 10 can provide a quick estimate of the beats per minute.

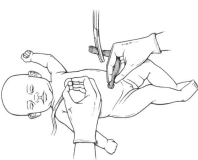

Figure 2.8. Determining heart rate by palpating base of cord and listening with a stethoscope

• *Color*

The baby should have pink lips and a pink trunk. Once adequate heart rate and ventilation are established, there should not be *central cyanosis*, which indicates hypoxemia.

What do you do if respirations or heart rate are abnormal?

 The most effective and important action in resuscitating a compromised newborn is to assist ventilation.

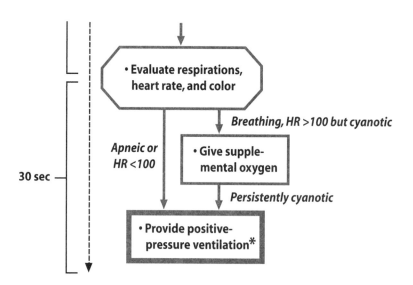

* Endotracheal intubation may become necessary if positive-pressure delivered by mask is not successful.

No matter which vital sign is abnormal, almost all compromised newborns respond to establishment or improvement of ventilation. Take a few seconds to minimize heat loss, clear the airway, and try to stimulate spontaneous respirations. If the baby is still apneic, the next appropriate action is to assist ventilation. This is accomplished by providing positive pressure to the airway with a bag and mask or T-piece resuscitator, as described in Lesson 3.

Remember, the entire resuscitation process up to this point should take no more than 30 seconds (or perhaps a bit longer if suctioning of meconium from the trachea was required).

 Administering free-flow oxygen or continuing to provide tactile stimulation to a nonbreathing newborn or to a newborn whose heart rate is less than 100 bpm is of little or no value and only delays appropriate treatment.

What do you do if the baby is breathing but has central cyanosis?

A baby's skin color, changing from blue to pink, can provide the most rapid and visible indicator of adequate breathing and circulation. The baby's skin color is best determined by looking at the central part of the body. Cyanosis caused by too little oxygen in the blood will appear as a blue hue to the lips, tongue, and central trunk. Healthy newborns sometimes have central cyanosis, but then become pink within a few seconds after birth. Even babies whose skin will eventually become heavily pigmented will appear "pink" when adequately oxygenated after birth. Acrocyanosis, which is a blue hue to only the hands and feet, may persist longer. Acrocyanosis without central cyanosis does not generally indicate that the baby's blood oxygen level is low and should not, by itself, be treated with oxygen. **Only central cyanosis requires intervention.** Turn to Center Page A to see color pictures of central cyanosis versus acrocyanosis (Figures A-2 and A-4).

If the baby is breathing but appears blue, administration of supplemental oxygen is indicated. Supplemental oxygen also may be needed when respirations are being assisted with a bag and mask or a T-piece resuscitator, as described in Lesson 3.*

*Note: there is some evidence that resuscitation with air (21% oxygen) is as effective as resuscitation with 100% oxygen. Until more evidence is available, this program will continue to recommend administering supplemental oxygen whenever a baby requiring resuscitation is cyanotic or whenever positive-pressure ventilation is required to restore a normal heart rate. This controversy will be discussed further in Lessons 3 and 8.

> See page A in the center of the book for color photographs of central cyanosis and acrocyanosis.

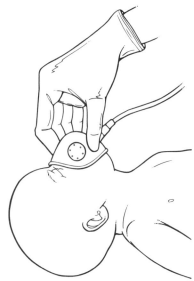

Figure 2.9. Oxygen mask held close to the baby's face to give close to 100% oxygen

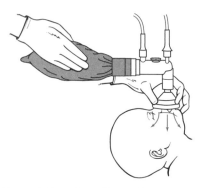

Figure 2.10. Using a flow-inflating bag to deliver free-flow oxygen. Hold the mask close to the face, but not so tight that pressure builds up

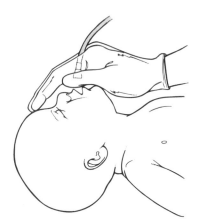

Figure 2.11. Oxygen delivered by tubing held in cupped hand over baby's face

• *Give supplemental oxygen*

Supplemental oxygen is not routinely needed at the beginning of a resuscitation. However, when a baby is cyanotic during resuscitation, the cyanosis may be relieved more quickly by administering a high concentration of oxygen. Your wall or portable oxygen source sends 100% oxygen through the tubing. As oxygen flows out of the tubing or mask, it mixes with room air, which contains only 21% oxygen. The concentration of oxygen that reaches the baby's nose is determined by the amount of 100% oxygen coming from the tube or mask (usually at least 5 L/min) and the amount of room air it must pass through to reach the baby. The closer the mask is to the face, the higher the concentration of oxygen breathed by the baby (Figure 2.9).

Free-flow oxygen refers to blowing oxygen over the baby's nose so that the baby breathes oxygen-enriched air. This can be accomplished by using one of the following delivery methods for a brief period:

• Oxygen mask

• *Flow*-inflating bag and mask

• T-piece resuscitator

• Oxygen tubing

A high concentration of free-flow oxygen is achieved most reliably with an oxygen mask, a flow-inflating resuscitation bag and mask, or a T-piece resuscitator, which you will learn about in Lesson 3. Whichever method you use, the mask should be held close to the face to keep the concentration of oxygen as high as possible, but not so tight that pressure builds up within the mask (Figures 2.9 and 2.10).

 Free-flow oxygen cannot be given reliably by a mask attached to a *self*-inflating bag. (See Lesson 3.)

If a mask is not immediately available, try to keep the oxygen concentrated around the baby's airway by using a funnel or by cupping your hand around the baby's face and the oxygen tubing (Figure 2.11).

If the baby continues to require supplemental oxygen, how should it be given?

After the resuscitation, when respirations and heart rate are stable and you have established that the newborn requires ongoing supplemental oxygen, pulse oximetry and arterial blood gas determinations should guide the appropriate oxygen concentration. Premature babies are particularly vulnerable to injury from excess oxygen. In Lesson 8 you will learn that use of blended oxygen and oximetry are recommended for adjusting the oxygen concentration when resuscitating babies born significantly preterm.

Oxygen that comes from a compressed source in the wall or from a tank is very cold and dry. To prevent heat loss and drying of the respiratory mucosa, oxygen given to newborns for long periods should be heated and humidified. However, during resuscitation, dry, unheated oxygen may be given for the few minutes required to stabilize the newborn's condition.

Avoid giving unheated and unhumidified oxygen at high flow rates (above approximately 10 L/min), because convective heat loss can become a significant problem. A flow rate of 5 L/min is usually adequate for free-flow oxygen during a resuscitation.

How do you know when to stop giving oxygen?

When the newborn no longer has central cyanosis, gradually withdraw the supplemental oxygen until the newborn can remain pink while breathing room air, or wean the oxygen as indicated by pulse oximetry.

Newborns who become cyanotic as supplemental oxygen is withdrawn should continue to receive enough oxygen to eliminate the blue hue to the lips, tongue, and central trunk. As soon as possible, arterial blood gas determinations and oximetry should be used to adjust oxygen levels to the normal range.

If cyanosis persists despite administration of free-flow oxygen, the baby may have significant lung disease, and a trial of positive-pressure ventilation may be indicated. (See Lesson 3.) If ventilation is adequate and the baby remains cyanotic, a diagnosis of cyanotic congenital heart disease or persistent pulmonary hypertension of the newborn should be considered. (See Lesson 7.)

Review

(The answers are in the preceding section and at the end of the lesson.)

11. A newborn is breathing and cyanotic. Your initial steps are to
    (Check all that are appropriate.)

    _____ Place the newborn on a radiant warmer.

    _____ Remove all wet linen.

    _____ Suction his mouth and nose.

    _____ Give free-flow oxygen.

    _____ Dry and stimulate.

12. Which drawings show the correct way to give free-flow oxygen to a baby who is cyanotic but is breathing well?

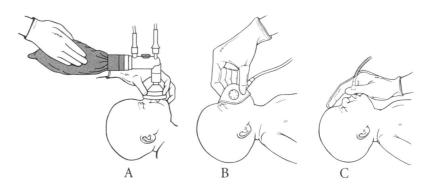

A   B   C

Key Points

1. If meconium is present and the newborn *is not vigorous,* suction the baby's trachea before proceeding with any other steps. If the newborn *is vigorous,* suction the mouth and nose only, and proceed with resuscitation as required.

2. "Vigorous" is defined as a newborn who has strong respiratory efforts, good muscle tone, and a heart rate greater than 100 beats per minute.

3. Open the airway by positioning the newborn in a "sniffing" position.

4. Appropriate forms of tactile stimulation are
   - Slapping or flicking the soles of the feet
   - Gently rubbing the back

5. Continued use of tactile stimulation in an apneic newborn wastes valuable time. For persistent apnea, begin positive-pressure ventilation promptly.

6. Free-flow oxygen is indicated for central cyanosis. Acceptable methods for administering free-flow oxygen are
   - Oxygen mask held firmly over the baby's face
   - Mask from a flow-inflating bag or T-piece resuscitator held closely over the baby's mouth and nose
   - Oxygen tubing cupped closely over the baby's mouth and nose

7. Free-flow oxygen cannot be given reliably by a mask attached to a self-inflating bag.

8. Decisions and actions during newborn resuscitation are based on the newborn's
   - Respirations   • Heart rate   • Color

9. Determine a newborn's heart rate by counting how many beats are in 6 seconds, then multiply by 10. For example, if you count 8 beats in 6 seconds, announce the baby's heart rate as 80 beats per minute.

Lesson 2 Review

(The answers follow.)

1. A newborn who is born at term, has no meconium in the amniotic fluid or on the skin, is breathing well, and has good muscle tone (does) (does not) need resuscitation.

2. A newborn with meconium in the amniotic fluid and who **is not vigorous** (will) (will not) need to have a laryngoscope inserted and be suctioned with an endotracheal tube.
   A newborn with meconium in the amniotic fluid and who **is vigorous** (will) (will not) need to have a laryngoscope inserted and be suctioned with an endotracheal tube.

3. When deciding which babies need tracheal suctioning, the term "vigorous" is defined by what 3 characteristics?

   (1)_____

   (2)_____

   (3)_____

4. When a suction catheter is used to clear the oropharynx of meconium before inserting an endotracheal tube, the appropriate size is _____F or_____F.

5. Which drawing shows the correct way to position a newborn's head prior to suctioning the airway?

   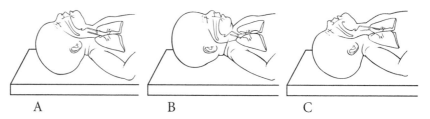

   A   B   C

6. A newborn is covered with meconium, is breathing well, has normal muscle tone, has a heart rate of 120 beats per minute, and is pink. The correct action is to

   _____ Insert a laryngoscope and suction his trachea with an endotracheal tube.

   _____ Suction the mouth and nose with a bulb syringe or suction catheter.

Lesson 2 Review — *continued*

7. In suctioning a baby's nose and mouth, the rule is to first suction
   the _____ and then
   the _____.

8. Make a check mark next to the correct ways to stimulate a
   newborn.

   _____ Slap on the back   _____ Slap on the sole of foot

   _____ Rub the back   _____ Squeeze the rib cage

9. If a baby is in secondary apnea, stimulation alone
   (will) (will not) stimulate breathing.

10. A newborn is still not breathing after a few seconds of stimulation.
    The next action should be to administer

    _____ Additional stimulation

    _____ Positive-pressure ventilation

11. A newborn is breathing and cyanotic. Your initial steps are to
    (Check all that are appropriate.)

    _____ Place the newborn on a radiant warmer.

    _____ Remove all wet linen.

    _____ Suction his mouth and nose.

    _____ Give free-flow oxygen.

    _____ Dry and stimulate.

12. Which drawings show the correct way to give free-flow oxygen to a
    baby who is cyanotic but is breathing well?

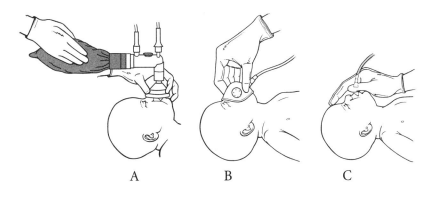

       A   B   C

Lesson 2 Review — *continued*

13. If you need to give oxygen for longer than a few minutes, the oxygen should be _____ and _____.

14. You have stimulated a newborn and suctioned her mouth. It is now 30 seconds after birth, and she is still apneic and pale. Her heart rate is 80 beats per minute. Your next action is to

    _____ Continue stimulation and give free-flow oxygen.

    _____ Provide positive-pressure ventilation.

15. You count a newborn's heartbeats for 6 seconds and count 6 beats. You report the heart rate as _____.

Answers to Questions

1. **Does not** need resuscitation.

2. A newborn with meconium who is not vigorous **will** need to have a laryngoscope inserted and be suctioned with an endotracheal tube. A newborn with meconium who is vigorous **will not** need to have a laryngoscope inserted and be suctioned with an endotracheal tube.

3. "Vigorous" is defined as: (1) **strong respiratory efforts,** (2) **good muscle tone,** and (3) **heart rate greater than 100 beats per minute.**

4. A **12F** or **14F** suction catheter should be used to suction meconium.

5. Correct head position is **A.**

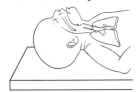

6. Since the newborn is active, he does not need to have his trachea suctioned, but you should **suction the mouth and nose with a bulb syringe or suction catheter.**

7. First suction the **mouth** and then the **nose.**

8. Stimulate by **slapping the sole of the foot** and/or **rubbing the back.**

9. Stimulation alone **will not** stimulate breathing if the baby is in secondary apnea.

10. If not breathing after stimulation, provide **positive-pressure ventilation.**

11. **All actions are indicated.**

12. **All drawings are correct.**

13. The oxygen should be **warmed** and **humidified.**

14. She should receive **positive-pressure ventilation.**

15. If you count 6 heartbeats in 6 seconds, report the baby's heart rate as **60 beats per minute (6 x 10 = 60).**

Performance Checklist
Lesson 2 — Initial Steps in Resuscitation

Instructor: The participant should be instructed to talk through the procedure as it is demonstrated. Judge the performance of each step and check (✓) the box when the action is completed correctly. If a step is done incorrectly, circle the box so that you can discuss that step later. You will need to provide information at several points concerning the condition of the baby.

Learner: To successfully complete this checklist, you should be able to perform all the steps and make all the correct decisions in the procedure. You should talk through the procedure as you perform it.

Equipment and Supplies
Newborn resuscitation manikin
Radiant warmer or table to simulate
	warmer
Gloves (or may simulate this)
Bulb syringe or suction catheter
Stethoscope
Shoulder roll
Blanket or towel to dry newborn
Self-inflating bag
	or
Flow-inflating bag with pressure
	manometer and oxygen source
	or
T-piece resuscitator
Flowmeter (or may simulate this)
Masks (term and preterm sizes)
Method to administer free-flow oxygen
	(oxygen mask, oxygen tubing,
	flow-inflating bag and mask, or
	T-piece resuscitator)
Laryngoscope and blade
Suction catheter
Endotracheal tube
Meconium aspirator
Clock with second hand
Mechanical suction and tubing
	(or may simulate this)

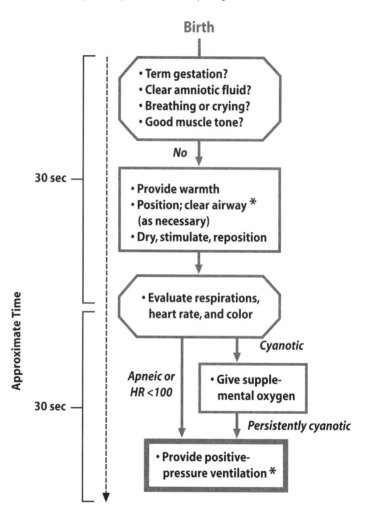

* Endotracheal intubation may be considered at several steps.

Performance Checklist

Lesson 2 — Initial Steps in Resuscitation

Name _____ Instructor _____ Date _____

Instructor's questions are in quotes. Learner's questions and correct responses are in bold type. Instructor should check boxes as the learner answers correctly.

"A newborn has just been born. Demonstrate how you would evaluate and care for this newborn. You may ask me any questions you would like to know about the newborn's condition as you progress."

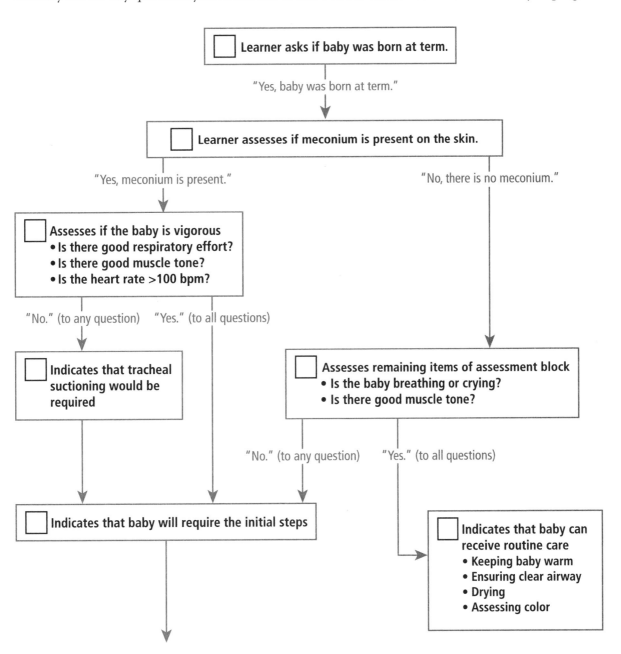

Initial Steps

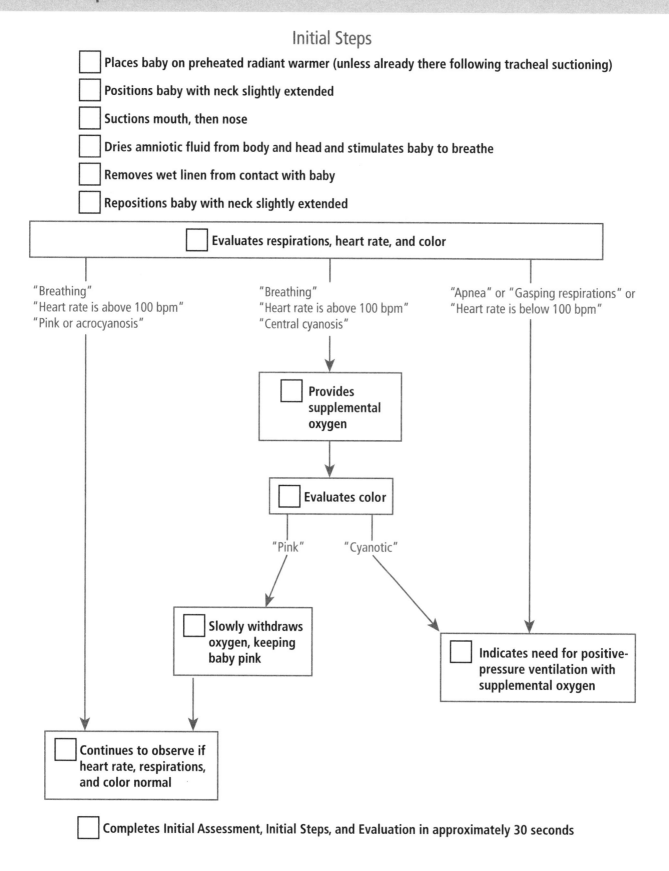

☐ Places baby on preheated radiant warmer (unless already there following tracheal suctioning)

☐ Positions baby with neck slightly extended

☐ Suctions mouth, then nose

☐ Dries amniotic fluid from body and head and stimulates baby to breathe

☐ Removes wet linen from contact with baby

☐ Repositions baby with neck slightly extended

☐ Evaluates respirations, heart rate, and color

"Breathing"
"Heart rate is above 100 bpm"
"Pink or acrocyanosis"

"Breathing"
"Heart rate is above 100 bpm"
"Central cyanosis"

"Apnea" or "Gasping respirations" or
"Heart rate is below 100 bpm"

☐ Provides supplemental oxygen

☐ Evaluates color

"Pink"   "Cyanotic"

☐ Slowly withdraws oxygen, keeping baby pink

☐ Indicates need for positive-pressure ventilation with supplemental oxygen

☐ Continues to observe if heart rate, respirations, and color normal

☐ Completes Initial Assessment, Initial Steps, and Evaluation in approximately 30 seconds

Use of Resuscitation Devices for Positive-Pressure Ventilation

In Lesson 3 you will learn

- When to give positive-pressure ventilation

- The similarities and differences among *flow-inflating bags, self-inflating bags,* and *T-piece resuscitators*

- The operation of each device to provide positive-pressure ventilation

- The correct placement of masks on the newborn's face

- How to test and troubleshoot devices used to provide positive-pressure ventilation

- How to evaluate the success of positive-pressure ventilation

The following case is an example of how to provide positive-pressure ventilation during resuscitation. As you read the case, imagine yourself as part of the resuscitation team. The details of how to deliver positive-pressure ventilation are then described in the remainder of the lesson.

Case 3.
Resuscitation with bag and mask and oxygen

A 20-year-old woman with pregnancy-induced hypertension has labor induced at 37 weeks' gestation. Several late decelerations of fetal heart rate are noted, but labor progresses quickly and a baby boy soon delivers.

He is apneic and limp and is taken to the radiant warmer, where the resuscitation team appropriately positions his head to open his airway, while his mouth and nose are cleared of secretions with a bulb syringe. He is dried with warmed towels, wet linen is removed, his head is repositioned, and he is further stimulated to breathe by flicking the soles of his feet.

No spontaneous respirations are noted after these stimulation activities and he has central cyanosis. He is then given positive-pressure ventilation with a bag and mask, using supplemental oxygen. A second person comes to assist and monitors the heart rate and breath sounds. The heart rate was initially 70 beats per minute (bpm). It increases as the positive-pressure ventilation continues.

After 30 seconds of positive-pressure ventilation, he remains apneic; however, his heart rate is reported to be 120 bpm. After another 30 seconds, he begins to breathe spontaneously. Positive-pressure ventilation is discontinued as spontaneous breathing normalizes. Supplemental oxygen is gradually reduced as the cyanosis resolves.

Several minutes after birth, the baby is breathing regularly, has a heart rate of 150 bpm, and remains pink without supplemental oxygen. He is shown to his mother, and his mother is encouraged to touch him while the next steps are explained. After a few more minutes of observation, the baby is moved to the nursery for post-resuscitation care, where vital signs and activity are monitored closely for deterioration.

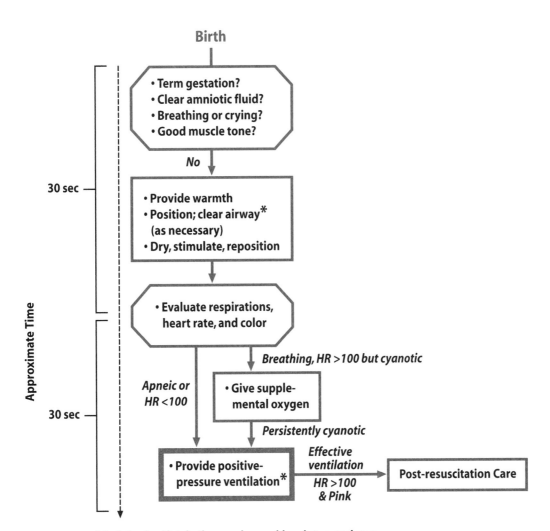

Birth

• Term gestation?
• Clear amniotic fluid?
• Breathing or crying?
• Good muscle tone?

No

• Provide warmth
• Position; clear airway*
  (as necessary)
• Dry, stimulate, reposition

• Evaluate respirations,
  heart rate, and color

Breathing, HR >100 but cyanotic

*Apneic or
HR <100*

• Give supple-
  mental oxygen

Persistently cyanotic

• Provide positive-
  pressure ventilation*

*Effective
ventilation
HR >100
& Pink*

Post-resuscitation Care

30 sec

Approximate Time

30 sec

* Endotracheal intubation may be considered at several steps.

What will this lesson cover?

In this lesson you will learn how to prepare and use a resuscitation bag and mask or a T-piece resuscitator to deliver positive-pressure ventilation.

You learned in Lesson 2 how to determine within a few seconds whether some form of resuscitation is required and how to perform the initial steps of resuscitation.

You begin resuscitation by minimizing heat loss; positioning; clearing the airway; stimulating the baby to breathe by drying as you reposition the head; and assessing respirations, heart rate, and color. If the baby is breathing but has central cyanosis, you administer free-flow supplemental oxygen.

If the baby is not breathing or is gasping, the heart rate is less than 100 bpm, and/or the color remains cyanotic despite supplemental oxygen, the next step is to provide positive-pressure ventilation.

! Ventilation of the lungs is the single most important and most effective step in cardiopulmonary resuscitation of the compromised newborn baby.

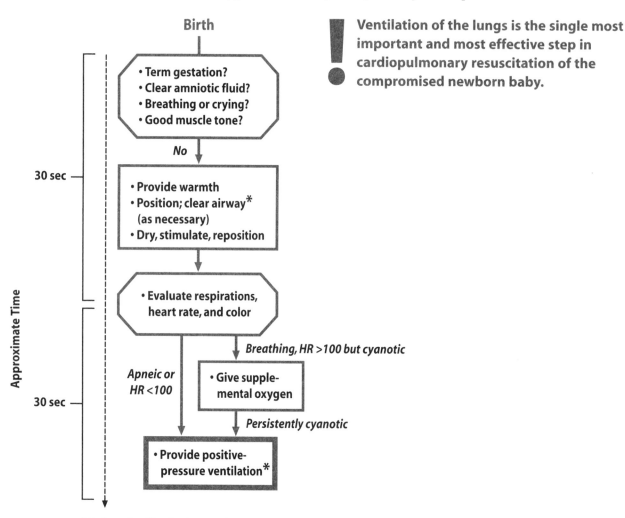

* Endotracheal intubation may be considered at several steps.

What are the different types of resuscitation devices available to ventilate newborns?

Three types of devices are available to ventilate newborns, and they work in different ways.

1. The *self-inflating bag* fills spontaneously after it is squeezed, pulling gas (oxygen or air or a mixture of both) into the bag.

2. The *flow-inflating bag* (also called an anesthesia bag) fills only when gas from a compressed source flows into it.

3. The *T-piece resuscitator* also works only when gas from a compressed source flows into it. The gas is directed either to the environment or to the baby by occluding or releasing the opening on a T-shaped tube with your finger or thumb.

Find out what kind of resuscitation device is used in your hospital. If your hospital uses the T-piece resuscitator in the delivery area, you should still learn the details of whichever of the 2 types of bags are commonly used outside of the delivery area. A self-inflating bag should be available as a backup wherever resuscitation may be needed, in case a compressed gas source fails or the T-piece device malfunctions. Details of all 3 of the devices are found in the Appendix to this lesson. You should read those section(s) of the Appendix that apply to the device(s) used in your hospital.

The *self-inflating bag,* as its name implies, inflates automatically without a compressed gas source (Figure 3.1). It remains inflated at all times, unless being squeezed. Peak inspiratory pressure (PIP) (or peak inflation pressure) is controlled by how hard the bag is squeezed. Positive end-expiratory pressure (PEEP) can be administered only if an additional valve is attached to the self-inflating bag. Continuous positive airway pressure (CPAP) while a patient is breathing spontaneously cannot be delivered reliably with a self-inflating bag. (Both PEEP and CPAP will be covered in more detail in Lesson 8.)

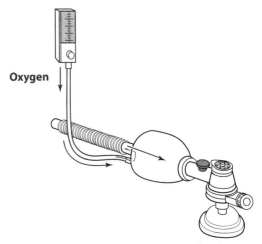

Oxygen

Figure 3.1. Self-inflating bag remains inflated without gas flow and without having the mask sealed on the face. An oxygen line is shown attached since supplemental oxygen is recommended whenever positive pressure is required

The **flow-inflating bag** is collapsed like a deflated balloon when not in use (Figure 3.2). It inflates only when a gas source is forced into the bag and the opening of the bag is sealed, as when the mask is placed tightly on a baby's face. Peak inspiratory pressure is controlled by the flow rate of incoming gas, adjustment of the flow-control valve, and how hard the bag is squeezed. Positive end-expiratory pressure (PEEP) (or CPAP) is controlled by an adjustable flow-control valve.

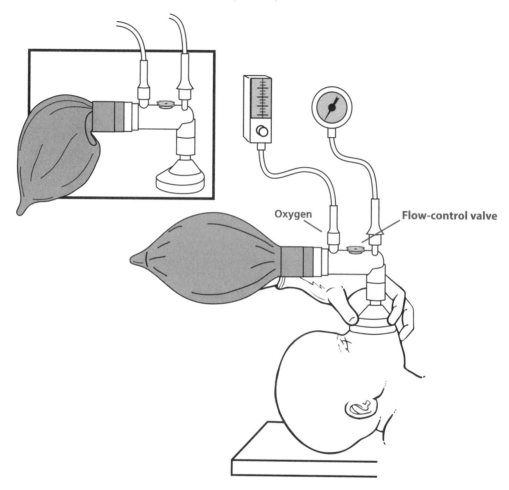

Oxygen Flow-control valve

Figure 3.2. Flow-inflating bag inflates only with a compressed gas source and with mask sealed on face; otherwise, the bag remains deflated (inset)

The *T-piece resuscitator* (Figure 3.3) is flow controlled and pressure limited. Like the flow-inflating bag, this device requires a compressed gas source. Peak inspiratory pressure and positive end-expiratory pressure (PEEP) (or CPAP), if desired, are set manually with adjustable controls. Intermittent inflation pressure is delivered when the operator alternately occludes and releases an opening on the device.

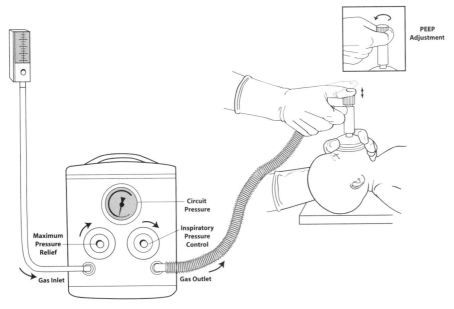

PEEP
Adjustment

Circuit
Pressure

Inspiratory
Pressure
Control

Maximum
Pressure
Relief

Gas Inlet

Gas Outlet

Figure 3.3. Flow-controlled, pressure-limited device (T-piece resuscitator). Pressures are pre-set by adjusting controls on the device and are delivered by occluding or releasing an opening behind the mask

What are the advantages and disadvantages of each assisted-ventilation device?

The *self-inflating bag* (Figure 3.4) is found more commonly in the hospital delivery room and resuscitation cart than the flow-inflating bag. It often is considered easier to use because it refills after being squeezed; this happens even if it is not attached to a compressed gas source and even if its mask is not on a patient's face. The disadvantage of this is that you will be less likely to know if you have achieved a good seal between the mask and the baby's face, which is required for the pressure from the squeezed bag to result in effective gas flow delivered to the baby's lungs.

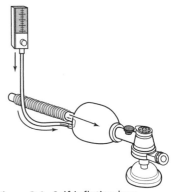

Figure 3.4. Self-inflating bag

Advantages
- Will always refill after being squeezed, even with no compressed gas source
- Pressure-release valve makes overinflation less likely

Disadvantages
- Will inflate even if there is not a seal between the mask and the patient's face
- Requires oxygen reservoir to provide high concentration of oxygen
- Cannot be used to deliver free-flow oxygen reliably through the mask
- Cannot be used to deliver continuous positive airway pressure (CPAP) and can deliver positive end-expiratory pressure (PEEP) only when a PEEP valve is added

When a self-inflating bag is not being squeezed, the amount of gas or oxygen flow that comes out of the patient outlet depends on the relative resistance and leaks in valves within the bag. Even when the self-inflating bag is connected to a 100% oxygen source, most of the oxygen is directed out of the back of the bag and an unpredictable amount is directed toward the patient unless the bag is being squeezed. Therefore, the self-inflating bag cannot be used to reliably deliver 100% free-flow oxygen through the mask. Also, as was described in Lesson 2, the self-inflating bag must have an oxygen reservoir attached to deliver a high concentration of oxygen, even when the bag is being squeezed.

Some neonatologists recommend administering CPAP to a spontaneously breathing baby, and PEEP to a baby who is receiving positive-pressure ventilation, particularly if the baby is born preterm. (See Lesson 8.) Continuous positive airway pressure cannot be administered effectively with a self-inflating bag, and PEEP can be delivered only if a special "PEEP valve" is used.

As a safety precaution, most self-inflating bags have a pressure release valve (pop-off valve) that limits the peak inspiratory pressure that can be delivered. If a self-inflating bag does not have a pressure release valve, then a gauge is needed to monitor peak inspiratory pressure.

The *flow-inflating bag* (Figure 3.5) requires a compressed gas source for inflation. When the gas flows into the device, it will take the path of least resistance and either flow out the patient outlet or into the bag. To make the bag inflate, you need to keep the gas from escaping by having the face mask sealed tightly against the newborn's face. Therefore, when a newborn is being resuscitated, the bag will not fill unless there is gas flow and the mask is tightly sealed over the baby's mouth and nose. Absent or partial inflation of the flow-inflating bag indicates that a tight seal has not been established.

In addition, because the oxygen concentration that exits a flow-inflating bag is the same as that which enters the bag, the flow-inflating bag can be used to deliver free-flow oxygen reliably at 21% to 100% concentration.

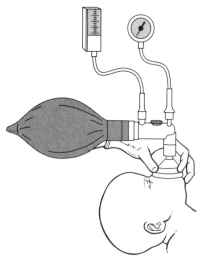

Figure 3.5. Flow-inflating bag
Advantages
- Delivers 21%–100% oxygen, depending on the source
- Easy to determine when there is a seal on the patient's face
- Can be used to deliver free-flow oxygen of 21%–100%

Disadvantages
- Requires a tight seal between the mask and the patient's face to remain inflated
- Requires a gas source to inflate
- Usually does not have a safety pop-off valve

The main disadvantage of using a flow-inflating bag is that it takes more practice to use effectively. Also, because it requires a gas source to inflate, it is sometimes not as quickly available for use when the need for resuscitation is unanticipated.

Because most flow-inflating bags do not have a safety valve, it is important to watch for change in heart rate, color, and degree of chest movement to avoid overinflation of the lungs. Checking the pressure gauge occasionally will be helpful to maintain consistency of each assisted breath.

The ***T-piece resuscitator*** (Figure 3.6) has many similarities to the flow-inflating bag, with the added safety of mechanically limiting airway pressures. Like the flow-inflating bag, the T-piece resuscitator requires gas flow from a compressed gas source and has an adjustable flow-control valve to regulate the desired amount of CPAP or PEEP. The T-piece resuscitator also requires a tight face-mask seal to deliver a breath and can reliably deliver 21% to 100% free-flow oxygen. The device also requires some preparation time to assemble it, turn on gas flow, and adjust the pressure limits appropriately for the expected needs of the newborn.

The T-piece resuscitator differs from the flow-inflating bag in that the peak inspiratory pressure is regulated by a mechanical adjustment instead of by the amount of squeeze on the bag. The T-piece resuscitator provides more consistent pressure and the operator is not subject to fatigue from squeezing the bag. Gas flow is directed to the baby or the environment when you alternately occlude and open the PEEP cap with your finger or thumb.

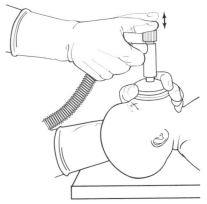

Figure 3.6. T-piece resuscitator
Advantages
• Consistent pressure
• Reliable control of peak inspiratory pressure and positive end-expiratory pressure
• Reliable delivery of 100% oxygen
• Operator does not become fatigued from bagging
Disadvantages
• Requires gas supply
• Compliance of the lung cannot be "felt"
• Requires pressures to be set prior to use
• Changing inflation pressure during resuscitation is more difficult

You will learn to assess the baby for the most important signs of effective positive-pressure ventilation: a rapid rise in heart rate, improvement in color and muscle tone, presence of audible breath sounds heard with a stethoscope, and noting adequate chest movement. If you watch for these important signs, positive-pressure ventilation can be provided quite effectively with any of the positive-pressure devices described in this lesson.

Signs of Effective Positive-Pressure Ventilation
• Rapid rise in heart rate
• Improvement in color and tone
• Audible breath sounds
• Chest movement

What are important characteristics of resuscitation devices used to ventilate newborns?

The equipment should be specifically designed for newborns. Consideration should be given to the following:

Appropriately sized masks

A variety of mask sizes, appropriate for babies of different sizes, should be available at every delivery, because it may be difficult to determine the appropriate size before birth. The mask should cover the chin, mouth, and nose, but not the eyes, while still being small enough to create a tight seal on the face.

Capability to deliver a variable oxygen concentration up to 100%

This program recommends that babies who require positive-pressure ventilation at birth initially be ventilated with a high concentration of oxygen. This can be accomplished by attaching a 100% oxygen source to a self-inflating bag with an oxygen reservoir, a flow-inflating bag, or a T-piece resuscitator. High oxygen concentrations cannot be achieved with a self-inflating bag without a reservoir. Premature babies or babies requiring assisted ventilation for longer than several minutes should have the oxygen concentration reduced as the baby becomes pink or as oxygen saturation normalizes. This will require the ability to mix oxygen and air, which will require a source for both compressed air and oxygen and the use of an oxygen blender to deliver a variable oxygen concentration to the resuscitation bag or T-piece resuscitator. The use of oxygen will be discussed later in this lesson, and mixing of oxygen and air is described in Lesson 8.

Capability to control peak pressure, end-expiratory pressure, and inspiratory time

Establishing adequate ventilation is the most important step in resuscitating newborns. The amount of positive pressure required will vary by the state of the newborn's lungs, and delivery of excessive positive pressure can injure the lung. Positive end-expiratory pressure (PEEP) (or CPAP) may be helpful for ventilating babies with immature lungs, as will be discussed in Lesson 8. Self-inflating bags cannot deliver PEEP without the addition of a special PEEP valve. The presence of a pressure gauge can be helpful to monitor the amount of peak and end-expiratory pressures being given.

The duration of inspiratory time is one factor that contributes to inflating the lungs. Increasing the inspiratory time is accomplished by squeezing on the bag for a longer time or by keeping your finger on the PEEP cap of the T-piece resuscitator longer. The optimum inflation time to use during resuscitation of a newborn has not been determined.

Appropriately sized bag

Bags used for newborns should have a volume of 200 to 750 mL. Term newborns require only 15 to 25 mL with each ventilation (5 to 8 mL/kg). Bags larger than 750 mL, which are designed for older children and adults, make it difficult to provide such small volumes. Bags that are too small will not permit long inflation times.

Safety features

To minimize complications resulting from high ventilation pressures, resuscitation devices should have certain safety features to prevent or guard against inadvertent use of high pressures. These features will be different for each type of device.

What safety features prevent the pressure in the device from getting too high?

You will attach a resuscitation device to either a mask, which will be held tightly against the patient's face, or to an endotracheal tube, which will be in the patient's trachea. In either case, if you ventilate with high pressure and/or rate, the lungs could become overinflated, causing rupture of the alveoli and a resulting air leak, such as a pneumothorax.

Self-inflating bags should have a pressure-release valve (commonly called a *pop-off valve*) (Figure 3.7), which generally is set by the manufacturer to 30 to 40 cm H_2O. If peak inspiratory pressures greater than 30 to 40 cm H_2O are generated, the valve opens, limiting the pressure being transmitted to the newborn. There may be wide variation in the point at which a pressure-release valve opens. The make and age of the bag as well as the method with which it has been cleaned affect the opening pressure of the valve.

In some self-inflating bags, the pressure-release valve can be temporarily occluded or bypassed to allow higher pressures to be administered. This is usually not necessary, but can be done to ventilate a newborn's non-aerated lungs when the usual pressures are not effective, especially with the first few breaths. Care must be taken not to use excessive pressure during the first few ventilations while the pressure-release valve is bypassed. Many self-inflating bags also are equipped with a pressure gauge or a port to attach a pressure gauge, which allows you to monitor the peak inspiratory pressure as you squeeze the bag.

Flow-inflating bags have a flow-control valve (Figure 3.8), which can be adjusted to deliver the desired positive end-expiratory pressure. If the flow-control valve is adjusted incorrectly, it is possible to inadvertently overinflate the baby's lungs. The pressure manometer is used to avoid excessive pressures.

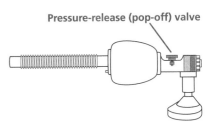

Figure 3.7. Self-inflating bag with pressure-release (pop-off) valve

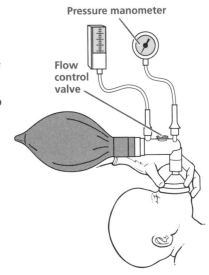

Figure 3.8. Flow-inflating bag with flow-control valve and pressure manometer

Be certain to connect the oxygen supply line to the correct connection site as indicated by the bag's manufacturer. Connection of the oxygen supply line to the pressure gauge port has been reported to result in inadvertent high-inflating pressures being delivered to the patient.

T-piece resuscitators have 2 controls to adjust the inspiratory pressure. The inspiratory pressure control sets the amount of pressure desired during a normal assisted breath. The maximum pressure relief control is a safety feature that prevents the pressure from exceeding a preset value (usually 40 cm H_2O, but adjustable). Excessive pressure also can be avoided by watching the circuit pressure gauge (Figure 3.9).

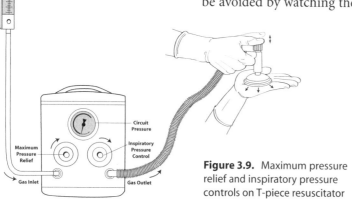

Figure 3.9. Maximum pressure relief and inspiratory pressure controls on T-piece resuscitator

Table 3-1. Controls of Respiratory Limits During Positive-Pressure Ventilation With Resuscitation Devices

Characteristic	Self-Inflating Bag	Flow-Inflating Bag	T-piece Resuscitator
Appropriate-sized Masks	Available	Available	Available
Oxygen Concentration: • 90%–100% capability • Variable concentration	• Only with reservoir • Only with blender plus reservoir • Approximately 40% O_2 delivered with no reservoir attached	• Yes • Only with blender	• Yes • Only with blender
Peak Inspiratory Pressure	Amount of squeeze measured by optional pressure gauge	Amount of squeeze measured by pressure gauge	Peak inspiratory pressure determined by adjustable mechanical setting
Positive End-expiratory Pressure (PEEP)	No direct control (unless optional PEEP valve attached)	Flow-control valve adjustment	Positive end-expiratory pressure control
Inspiratory Time	Duration of squeeze	Duration of squeeze	Duration that PEEP cap is occluded.
Appropriate-sized Bag	Available	Available	Not applicable
Safety Features	• Pop-off valve • Optional pressure gauge	• Pressure gauge	• Maximum pressure relief valve • Pressure gauge

Each of these characteristics will be described in the Appendix, under the detailed description of each device.

Review

(The answers are in the preceding section and at the end of the lesson.)

1. Flow-inflating bags (will) (will not) work without a compressed gas source.

2. A baby is born apneic and cyanotic. You clear his airway and stimulate him. Thirty seconds after birth, he has not improved. The next step is to (stimulate him more) (begin positive-pressure ventilation).

3. The single most important and most effective step in neonatal resuscitation is (stimulation) (ventilating the lungs).

4. Label these bags "flow-inflating," "self-inflating," or "T-piece resuscitator."

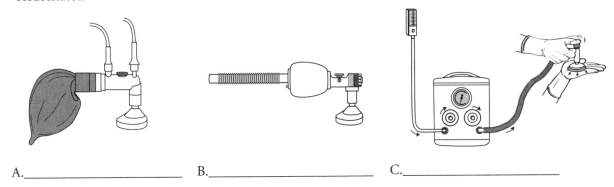

A._____   B._____   C._____

5. Masks of different sizes (do) (do not) need to be available at every delivery.

6. Self-inflating bags require the attachment of a(n) _____ to deliver 90% to 100% oxygen.

7. T-piece resuscitators (will) (will not) work without a compressed gas source.

8. Neonatal ventilation bags are (much smaller than) (the same size as) adult ventilation bags.

9. List the principal safety feature for each of the following devices:

   Self-inflating bag: _____

   Flow-inflating bag: _____

   T-piece resuscitator: _____

What concentration of oxygen should be used when giving positive-pressure ventilation during resuscitation?

This program recommends that 100% supplemental oxygen should be used when positive-pressure ventilation is required during resuscitation of term babies. Therefore, if you use a self-inflating bag, connect the bag to an oxygen source and use an oxygen reservoir. If you use a flow-inflating bag or T-piece resuscitator, connect these devices to an oxygen source.

Several recent studies suggest that resuscitation with 21% oxygen (room air) is just as successful as resuscitation with 100% oxygen. There is also some evidence that prolonged exposure to 100% oxygen during and following perinatal asphyxia may be harmful. However, since asphyxia involves deprivation of oxygen to body tissues and pulmonary blood flow is improved with oxygen, there is a theoretical possibility that using supplemental oxygen during resuscitation will result in more rapid restoration of tissue oxygen and, perhaps, less permanent tissue damage and improved blood flow to the lungs.

The currently available evidence is insufficient to resolve this controversy. Some clinicians will elect to start resuscitation using less than 100% oxygen, including some that will start with no supplemental oxygen (ie, room air). The evidence suggests that these approaches are reasonable in most circumstances. However, if one chooses to start resuscitation with room air, it is recommended that supplemental oxygen, up to 100%, be used if there is no appreciable improvement within 90 seconds following birth. There is clear agreement that ensuring effective ventilation should be the priority. Therefore, in situations where supplemental oxygen is not readily available, positive pressure should be administered with room air. The special circumstance of perhaps using less than 100% oxygen when resuscitating preterm babies will be covered in Lesson 8.

The American Academy of Pediatrics (AAP) and American Heart Association (AHA) acknowledge the developing evidence in this area and support the option of using less supplemental oxygen as described above. However, until further evidence to the contrary is available, this program continues to recommend using supplemental oxygen in the manner described in this textbook.

Can you give free-flow oxygen using a resuscitation device?

Free-flow oxygen cannot be given reliably through the mask of a self-inflating bag-and-mask device (Figure 3.10).

The oxygen flow entering a self-inflating bag will normally be diverted to the air inlet, through its attached oxygen reservoir, and then evacuated either out the end of the oxygen reservoir or out a valve that is attached to the reservoir. The amount of oxygen sent to the patient will depend on the relative resistance of the various valves and, therefore, may not reach the patient unless the bag is being squeezed. If your hospital is equipped with self-inflating bags, you may need to have a separate setup available for delivering free-flow oxygen, as described in Lesson 2.

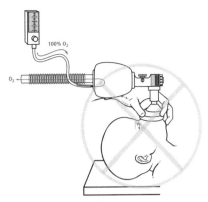

Figure 3.10. Free-flow 100% oxygen cannot be given reliably by self-inflating bag; bag must be squeezed for reliable 90% to 100% oxygen delivery

A flow-inflating bag or T-piece resuscitator can be used to deliver free-flow oxygen (Figure 3.11).

The mask should be loosely placed on the face, allowing some gas to escape around the edges. If the mask is held tightly to the face, pressure will build up in the bag or in the T-piece device and be transmitted to the newborn's lungs in the form of CPAP or PEEP. (See Lesson 8.) The bag should not inflate when used to provide free-flow oxygen. An inflated bag indicates that the mask is tight against the face and positive pressure is being provided.

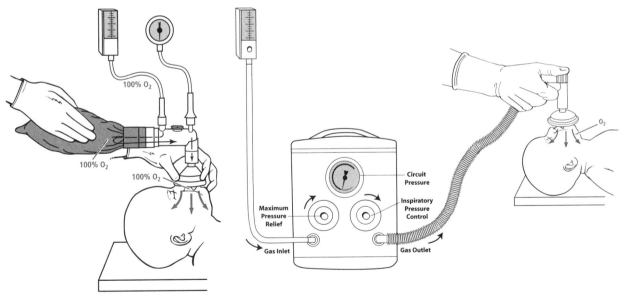

Figure 3.11. Free-flow oxygen given by flow-inflating bag (left) and by T-piece resuscitator (right). Note that mask is not held tightly on the face

What characteristics of face masks make them effective for ventilating newborns?

Masks come in a variety of shapes, sizes, and materials. Selection of a mask for use with a particular newborn depends on how well the mask fits and conforms to the newborn's face. The correct mask will achieve a tight seal between the mask and the newborn's face.

Resuscitation masks have rims that are either **cushioned** or **noncushioned.**

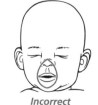

Figure 3.12. Face masks with cushioned rims

The rim on a *cushioned* mask (Figure 3.12) is made from either a soft, flexible material, such as foam rubber, or an air-inflated ring. A cushioned-rim mask has several advantages over a mask without a cushioned rim.

- The rim conforms more easily to the shape of the newborn's face, making it easier to form a seal.

- It requires less pressure on the newborn's face to obtain a seal.

- There is less chance of damaging the newborn's eyes if the mask is incorrectly positioned.

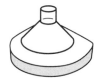

Figure 3.13. Round (left) and anatomically shaped (right) face masks

Some masks are constructed without a padded, soft rim. Such a mask usually has a very firm edge to the rim. A mask with a noncushioned rim can cause several problems.

- It is more difficult to obtain a seal, because it does not easily conform to the shape of the baby's face.

- It can damage the eyes if the mask is improperly positioned.

- It can bruise the newborn's face if the mask is applied too firmly.

Masks also come in 2 shapes: round and anatomically shaped (Figure 3.13). Anatomically shaped masks are shaped to fit the contours of the face. They are made to be placed on the face with the most pointed part of the mask fitting over the nose.

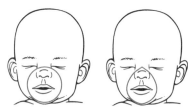

Correct
Covers mouth, nose, and chin but not eyes

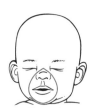

Incorrect
Too large: covers eyes and extends over chin

Incorrect
Too small: does not cover nose and mouth well

Figure 3.14. Correct (top) and incorrect (bottom) mask sizes

Masks also come in several sizes. Masks suitable for small premature babies as well as for term babies should be available for use.

For the mask to be the correct size, the rim will cover the tip of the chin, the mouth, and the nose, but not the eyes (Figure 3.14).

- Too large—may cause eye damage and will not seal well

- Too small—will not cover the mouth and nose and may occlude the nose

Be sure to have various-sized masks available. Effective ventilation of a preterm baby with a term-infant size mask is impossible.

How do you prepare the resuscitation device for an anticipated resuscitation?

Assemble the equipment

The positive-pressure ventilation device should be assembled and connected to an oxygen supply so that it can provide 90% to 100% concentration, if needed. If a self-inflating bag is used, be sure the oxygen reservoir is attached. Anticipate the size of the baby at delivery, and be sure you have appropriate-sized masks. Check the masks carefully for any cracks or defects in the rim. With each of the resuscitation devices, using an oxygen-air blender will facilitate adjustment of oxygen delivery after the initial resuscitation, although a blender is not essential to successfully resuscitate a newborn.

Test the equipment

Once the equipment has been selected and assembled, check the device and mask to be sure they function properly. Success in mask ventilation requires more than up-to-date equipment and a skilled operator—the equipment must be in working order. Bags that have cracks or holes, valves that stick or leak, devices that do not function properly, or defective masks must not be used. The equipment should be checked before each delivery. The operator should check it again just before its use. There are different things to check on each of the devices, as described in the respective appendices.

 Be very familiar with the type of resuscitation device(s) you are using. Know exactly how to check it to quickly determine whether it is functioning properly.

Review

(The answers are in the preceding section and at the end of the lesson.)

10. Free-flow oxygen can be delivered reliably through the mask attached to a (flow-inflating bag) (self-inflating bag) (T-piece resuscitator).

11. When giving free-flow oxygen with a flow-inflating bag and mask, it is necessary to place the mask (securely) (loosely) on the baby's face to allow some gas to escape around the edges of the mask.

12. Which mask is correct?

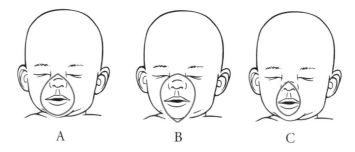

A   B   C

13. Before an anticipated resuscitation, the ventilation device should be connected to a(n) _____.

What do you need to check before beginning positive-pressure ventilation?

Select the appropriate-sized mask.
Remember, the mask should cover the mouth, nose, and tip of the chin, but not the eyes (Figure 3.15).

Be sure there is a clear airway.
You may want to suction the mouth and nose one more time to be certain there will be no obstruction to the assisted breaths that you will be delivering.

Position the baby's head.
As described in Lesson 2, the baby's neck should be slightly extended (but not overextended) into the "sniffing position" to maintain an open airway. One way to accomplish this is to place a small roll under the shoulders (Figure 3.16).

If the baby's position has shifted, reposition the baby before continuing.

Figure 3.15. Correct-sized mask covers mouth, nose, and tip of chin, but not the eyes

Figure 3.16. Correct position for assisted ventilation

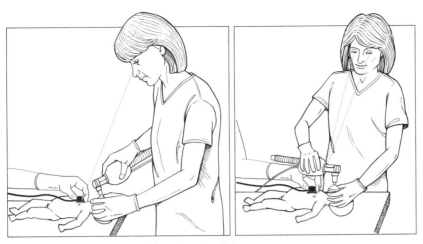

Figure 3.17. Two correct positions for visualizing chest movement during assisted ventilation

Position yourself at the bedside.

You also will need to position yourself at the baby's side or head to use a resuscitation device effectively (Figure 3.17). Both positions leave the chest and abdomen unobstructed for visual monitoring of the baby, for chest compressions, and for vascular access via the umbilical cord should these procedures become necessary. If you are right-handed, you probably will feel most comfortable controlling the resuscitation device with your right hand and the mask with your left hand. If you are left-handed, you probably will want to control the resuscitation device with your left hand and hold the mask with your right hand. The mask may be swiveled to orient it properly.

How do you position the mask on the face?

The mask should be placed on the face so that it covers the nose and mouth, and the tip of the chin rests within the rim of the mask. You may find it helpful to begin by cupping the chin in the mask and then covering the nose (Figure 3.18).

The mask usually is held on the face with the thumb, index, and/or middle finger encircling much of the rim of the mask, while the ring and fifth fingers lift the chin forward to maintain a patent airway.

Anatomically shaped masks should be positioned with the pointed end over the nose. Once the mask is positioned, an airtight seal can be formed by using light downward pressure on the rim of the mask and/or gently squeezing the mandible up toward the mask (Figure 3.19).

Care should be taken in holding the mask. Observe the following precautions:

- Do not "jam" the mask down on the face. Too much pressure can bruise the face.
- Be careful not to rest your fingers or hand on the baby's eyes.

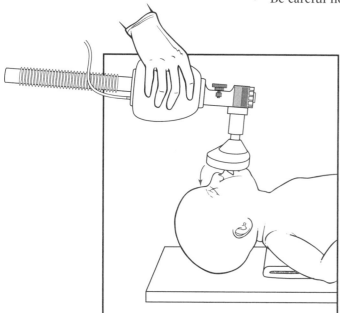

Figure 3.18. Correctly positioning mask on face

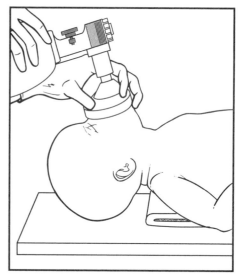

Figure 3.19. Light pressure on the mask will help create a seal. Anterior pressure on the posterior rim of the mandible (not shown) may also help

Why is establishing a seal between the mask and the face so important?

An airtight seal between the rim of the mask and the face is essential to achieve the positive pressure required to inflate the lungs *with any of the resuscitation devices.*

Although a self-inflating bag will remain inflated despite an inadequate seal, you will not be able to generate pressure to inflate the lungs when you squeeze the bag.

A flow-inflating bag will not inflate without a good mask-face seal and, therefore, you won't be able to squeeze the bag to create the desired pressure.

A T-piece resuscitator will not deliver positive pressure unless there is a good mask-face seal.

Remember

- A tight seal is required for a flow-inflating bag to inflate.
- A tight seal is required for each of the resuscitation devices to generate positive pressure to inflate the lungs.

How do you know how much inflation pressure to deliver?

 The best indication that the mask is sealed and the lungs are being adequately inflated is an improvement in heart rate, color, and muscle tone.

Rapid rise in the baby's heart rate and subsequent improvement in color and muscle tone are the best indicators that inflation pressures are adequate. If these signs are not improving, you should look for the presence of chest movement with each positive-pressure breath and have an assistant listen to both sides of the lateral areas of the chest with a stethoscope to assess breath sounds. Abdominal movement due to air entering the stomach may be mistaken for effective ventilation.

The lungs of a fetus are filled with fluid, but the lungs of a newborn must be filled with air. To establish a gaseous volume (functional residual capacity) in the lungs, the first few breaths often require higher pressure than subsequent breaths. This requirement for increased pressure is more likely to be found in a baby who is not breathing spontaneously.

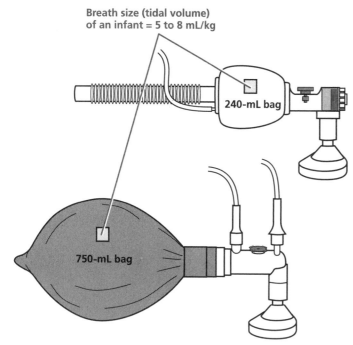

Breath size (tidal volume) of an infant = 5 to 8 mL/kg

240-mL bag

750-mL bag

Figure 3.20. Relative sizes of a normal breath and common resuscitation bags

High lung volumes and airway pressures may cause lung injury, so it is recommended to squeeze on the resuscitation bag just enough to improve heart rate, color, and muscle tone. Increasing the amount of positive pressure to 30 cm H_2O or greater is occasionally necessary if no improvement in these parameters occurs. It is helpful to monitor airway pressure with a pressure gauge to avoid high lung volumes and airway pressures, to assess compliance of the lungs and, if needed, to guide selection of subsequent ventilator settings.

If the baby appears to be taking very deep breaths, the lungs are being overinflated. You are using too much pressure, and there is danger of producing a pneumothorax.

Remember that the volume of a normal newborn breath is much smaller than the amount of gas in your resuscitation bag: one tenth of a 240-mL self-inflating bag; one thirtieth of a 750-mL flow-inflating bag (Figure 3.20).

What ventilation rate should you provide during positive-pressure ventilation?

During the initial stages of neonatal resuscitation, breaths should be delivered at a rate of **40 to 60 breaths per minute,** or slightly less than once a second.

To help maintain a rate of 40 to 60 breaths per minute, try saying the following to yourself as you ventilate the newborn:

Breathe . . . . Two . . . . Three . . . . Breathe . . . . Two . . . . Three . . . . .
(squeeze) (release . . . .) (squeeze) (release . . . .)

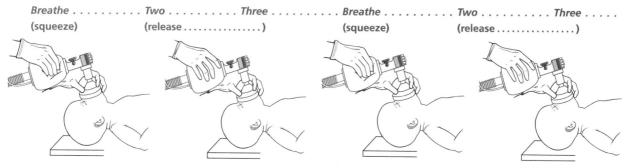

Figure 3.21. Counting out loud to maintain a rate of 40 to 60 breaths per minute

If you squeeze the bag or occlude the PEEP cap of the T-piece resuscitator on "Breathe," and release while you say "Two, Three," you will probably find you are ventilating at a proper rate (Figure 3.21).

How do you know if the baby is improving and that you can stop positive-pressure ventilation?

Improvement is indicated by the following 4 signs:

- Increasing heart rate
- Improving color
- Spontaneous breathing
- Improving muscle tone

Check the 4 signs for improvement after 30 seconds of administering positive pressure. This requires the assistance of another person. If the heart rate remains below 60 bpm, you need to proceed to the next step of chest compressions as described in the next lesson. But if the heart rate is above 60 bpm, you should continue to administer positive-pressure ventilation and assess the 4 signs every 30 seconds.

As the heart rate increases toward normal, continue ventilating the baby at a rate of 40 to 60 breaths per minute. With improvement, the baby also should become pink and muscle tone should improve. Monitor the movement of the chest and breath sounds to avoid overinflation or underinflation of the lungs.

When the heart rate stabilizes above 100 bpm, reduce the rate and pressure of assisted ventilation until you see effective spontaneous respirations. When color improves, supplemental oxygen also can be weaned as tolerated.

What do you do if the heart rate, color, and muscle tone do not improve and the baby's chest is not moving during positive-pressure ventilation?

If the heart rate, color, and muscle tone do not improve, check to see if the chest is moving with each positive-pressure breath and ask the second person to listen with a stethoscope for breath sounds. If the chest does not expand adequately and there are poor breath sounds, it may be due to one or more of the following reasons:

- The seal is inadequate.
- The airway is blocked.
- Not enough pressure is being given.

Inadequate seal

If you hear or feel air escaping from around the mask, reapply the mask to the face to form a better seal. Use a little more pressure on the rim of the mask and lift the jaw a little more forward. Do not press down hard on the baby's face. The most common place for a leak to occur is between the cheek and bridge of the nose (Figure 3.22).

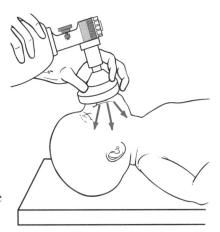

Figure 3.22. Inadequate seal of mask on face may result in poor chest rise

Blocked airway

Another possible reason for insufficient ventilation of the baby's lungs is a blocked airway. To correct this,

- Check the baby's position and extend the neck a bit farther.

- Check the mouth, oropharynx, and nose for secretions; suction the mouth and nose if necessary.

- Try ventilating with the baby's mouth slightly open (especially helpful in extremely small premature babies with very small nares).

Not enough pressure

You may be providing inadequate inspiratory pressure.

- Increase the pressure. If using a resuscitation device with a *pressure gauge,* note the amount of pressure required to achieve improvements in heart rate, color, tone, breath sounds, and perceptible chest movement.

- If using a bag with a *pressure-release valve,* increase the pressure until the valve actuates. If more pressure is required and it is possible to occlude the pressure-release valve, do so, and cautiously increase the pressure.

- If physiologic improvement still cannot be achieved, endotracheal intubation may be required.

In summary, if you do not observe physiologic improvement, check for chest movement. If there is no movement, try the following steps until the chest expands:

Conditions	Actions
1. Inadequate seal	Reapply mask to face and lift the jaw forward.
2. Blocked airway	Reposition the head. Check for secretions; suction if present. Ventilate with the newborn's mouth slightly open.
3. Not enough pressure	Increase pressure until there is a perceptible movement of the chest. Consider endotracheal intubation.

If you still are unable to obtain physiologic improvement and adequate chest movement after going through this sequence, endotracheal intubation and positive-pressure ventilation through the endotracheal tube are usually required.

Review

(The answers are in the preceding section and at the end of the lesson.)

14. Which baby is positioned properly for positive-pressure ventilation?

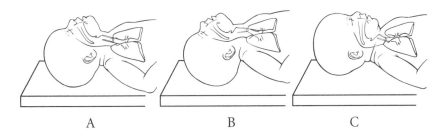

A   B   C

15. Which illustration(s) shows the correct position for assisting positive-pressure ventilation?

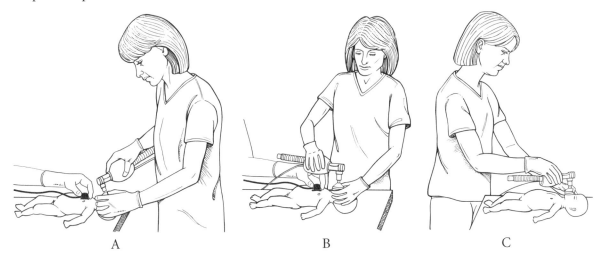

A   B   C

16. You must hold the resuscitation device so that you can see the newborn's _____ and _____.

17. An anatomically shaped mask should be positioned with the (pointed) (rounded) end over the newborn's nose.

18. If you notice that the baby's chest looks as if he is taking deep breaths, you are (overinflating) (underinflating) the lungs, and it is possible that a pneumothorax may occur.

19. When ventilating a baby, you should provide positive-pressure ventilation at a rate of _____ to _____ breaths per minute.

20. Before stopping assisted ventilation, you should note improvement in the following 4 physical signs:

    (1)_____

    (2)_____

    (3)_____

    (4)_____

21. You are using a self-inflating bag to ventilate a baby. The bag fills after every squeeze. The baby's heart rate, color, and muscle tone are not improving and there is no perceptible chest movement with each breath. List 3 possibilities of what may be wrong.

    (1)_____

    (2)_____

    (3)_____

22. If, after making appropriate adjustments, you are unable to obtain physiologic improvement and chest expansion with positive-pressure ventilation, you usually will have to insert a(n)

    _____.

23. You notice that a baby's heart rate, color, and muscle tone are improving and the baby's chest is moving as you provide positive-pressure ventilation. Another way to check for good aeration is to use a _____ to listen for _____ sounds in both lungs.

Is there anything else to do if positive-pressure ventilation with a mask is to be continued for more than several minutes?

Newborns requiring positive-pressure ventilation with a mask for longer than several minutes should have an orogastric tube inserted and left in place.

During positive-pressure ventilation with a mask, gas is forced into the oropharynx where it can enter both the trachea and the esophagus. Proper positioning of the newborn will transmit most of the air into the trachea and the lungs. However, some gas may enter the esophagus and be forced into the stomach (Figure 3.23).

Gas forced into the stomach interferes with ventilation in the following ways:

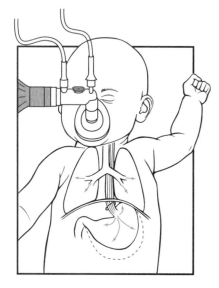

Figure 3.23. Excess gas in stomach resulting from bag-and-mask ventilation

- A stomach distended with gas puts upward pressure on the diaphragm, preventing full expansion of the lungs.

- Gas in the stomach may cause regurgitation of gastric contents, which may then be aspirated during positive-pressure ventilation.

The problems related to gastric/abdominal distention and aspiration of gastric contents can be reduced by inserting an orogastric tube, suctioning gastric contents, and leaving the gastric tube in place and uncapped, to act as a vent for stomach gas throughout the remainder of the resuscitation.

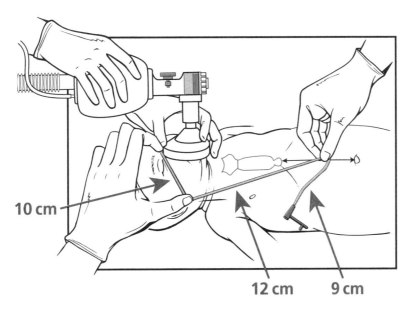

10 cm

12 cm   9 cm

Figure 3.24. Measuring the correct distance for inserting an orogastric tube

How do you insert an orogastric tube?

The equipment you will need to place an orogastric tube during ventilation includes

• 8F feeding tube

• 20-mL syringe

The major steps are as follows:

1. First measure the amount of tube you want to insert. It must be long enough to reach the stomach but not so long as to pass beyond it. The length of the inserted tube should be equal to *the distance from the bridge of the nose to the earlobe and from the earlobe to a point halfway between the xyphoid process* (the lower tip of the sternum) and the umbilicus. Note the centimeter mark at this place on the tube (Figure 3.24).

   To minimize interruption of ventilation, measurement of the orogastric tube can be approximated with the mask in place.

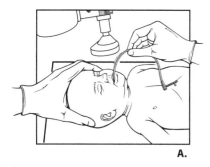

A.

2. Insert the tube through the **mouth** rather than the nose (Figure 3.25A). The nose should be left open for ventilation. Ventilation can be resumed as soon as the tube has been placed.

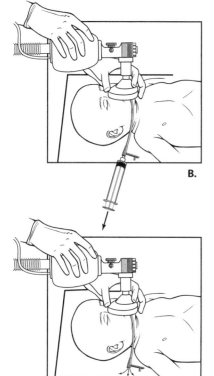

B.

3. Once the tube is inserted the desired distance, attach a syringe and quickly but gently remove the gastric contents (Figure 3.25B).

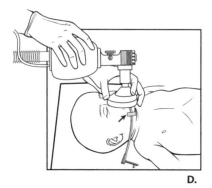

C.

4. Remove the syringe from the tube and leave the end of the tube *open* to provide a vent for air entering the stomach (Figure 3.25C).

D.

5. Tape the tube to the baby's cheek to ensure that the tip remains in the stomach and is not pulled back into the esophagus (Figure 3.25D).

Figure 3.25. Insertion, aspiration, and taping of an orogastric tube (top to bottom)

The tube will not interfere with the mask-to-face seal if an 8F feeding tube is used and the tube exits from the side of the mask over the soft area of the baby's cheek. A larger tube may make it difficult to obtain a seal, particularly in premature infants. A smaller tube can easily become occluded by secretions.

What do you do if the baby is *not* improving?

The vast majority of babies requiring resuscitation will improve if given adequate positive-pressure ventilation. Therefore, you should ensure that the lungs are being adequately ventilated with supplemental oxygen. If the baby still is not improving, consider the following:

Is chest movement adequate?

Check for adequacy of chest movement, and use a stethoscope to listen for bilateral breath sounds.

- Is the face-mask seal tight?
- Is the airway blocked because of improper head position or secretions in the nose, mouth, or pharynx?
- Is the resuscitation equipment working properly?
- Is adequate pressure being used?
- Is air in the stomach interfering with chest expansion?

Is adequate oxygen being administered?

- Is the oxygen tubing attached to the ventilation device *and* to the oxygen source?
- Is gas flowing through the flowmeter?
- If using a self-inflating bag, is the oxygen reservoir attached?
- If using a tank (rather than wall oxygen), is there oxygen in the tank?

These all seem obvious. However, in the atmosphere of urgency created by a newborn needing resuscitation, some of these points may be overlooked.

Positive-pressure ventilation with a mask generally is not as effective as positive-pressure ventilation through an endotracheal tube. A mask does not seal on the face as tightly as an endotracheal tube seals in the larynx. Also, with a mask, some of the positive pressure will escape down the esophagus into the stomach.

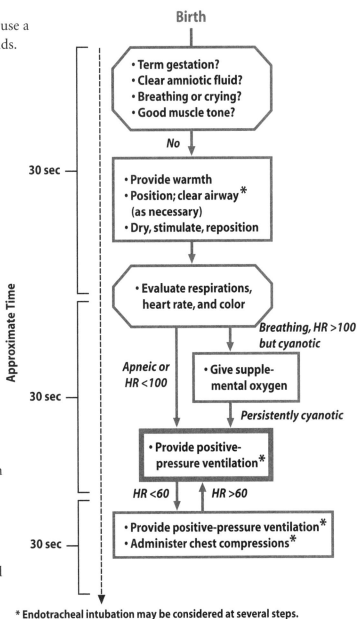

* Endotracheal intubation may be considered at several steps.

Therefore, if you have checked all of these factors and chest expansion is still not satisfactory, or if you don't hear good breath sounds bilaterally, it usually will be necessary to insert an endotracheal tube at this time. This procedure will be described in Lesson 5. If the baby has spontaneous but labored respirations, a brief trial of continuous positive airway pressure may be considered before inserting an endotracheal tube. The use of CPAP in preterm babies will be discussed in Lesson 8.

If a baby is not improving with assisted ventilation, other complications, such as a pneumothorax or hypovolemia, also may be present. These will be described in Lessons 6 and 7.

Establishing effective ventilation is the key to nearly all successful neonatal resuscitations.

If the baby's condition continues to deteriorate or fails to improve, and the heart rate is less than 60 bpm despite 30 seconds of adequate positive-pressure ventilation, your next step will be to begin chest compressions. This will be described in Lesson 4.

Review

(The answers are in the preceding section and at the end of the lesson.)

24. If you must continue positive-pressure ventilation with a mask for more than several minutes, a(n) _____ should be inserted to act as a vent for the gas in the stomach during the remainder of the resuscitation.

25. How far should this orogastric catheter be inserted? _____ cm

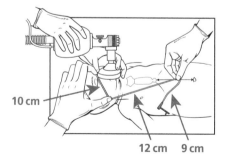

10 cm

12 cm   9 cm

26. As soon as the orogastric catheter is inserted, a syringe is attached and gastric contents are removed. Then the syringe is removed, and the catheter is left _____ to vent stomach gas.

27. The vast majority of babies requiring resuscitation (will) (will not) improve with positive-pressure ventilation.

Key Points

1. Ventilation of the lungs is the single most important and most effective step in cardiopulmonary resuscitation of the compromised newborn.

2. Indications for positive-pressure ventilation are
   - Apnea/gasping
   - Heart rate less than 100 beats per minute even if breathing
   - Persistent central cyanosis despite 100% free-flow oxygen

3. Self-inflating bags
   - Fill spontaneously after they are squeezed, pulling oxygen or air into the bag
   - Remain inflated at all times
   - Must have a tight face-mask seal to inflate the lungs
   - Can deliver positive-pressure ventilation without a compressed gas source; user must be certain the bag is connected to an oxygen source for the purpose of neonatal resuscitation
   - Require attachment of an oxygen reservoir to deliver 90% to 100% oxygen
   - Cannot be used to administer free-flow oxygen reliably through the mask

4. Flow-inflating bags
   - Fill only when gas from a compressed source flows into them
   - Depend on a compressed gas source
   - Must have a tight face-mask seal to inflate
   - Use a flow-control valve to regulate pressure/inflation
   - Look like a deflated balloon when not in use
   - Can be used to administer free-flow oxygen

5. The flow-inflating bag will not work if
   - The mask is not properly sealed over the newborn's nose and mouth.
   - There is a hole in the bag.
   - The flow-control valve is open too far.
   - The pressure gauge is missing or the port is not occluded.

Key Points — *continued*

6. T-piece resuscitators
   - Depend on a compressed gas source.
   - Must have a tight face-mask seal to inflate the lungs.
   - Operator sets maximum circuit pressure, peak inspiratory pressure, and positive end-expiratory pressure (PEEP).
   - Peak inspiratory pressure must be adjusted during resuscitation to achieve physiologic improvement, audible breath sounds, and perceptible chest movements.
   - Positive pressure is provided by alternately occluding and releasing the hole in the PEEP cap.
   - Can be used to deliver free-flow oxygen.

7. Every resuscitation device must have
   - A pressure release (pop-off) valve
   and/or
   - A pressure gauge and a flow-control valve

8. An oxygen reservoir must be attached to deliver high concentrations of oxygen using a self-inflating bag. Without the reservoir, the bag delivers only about 40% oxygen, which may be insufficient for neonatal resuscitation.

9. If there is no physiologic improvement and no perceptible chest expansion during assisted ventilation,
   - Reapply mask to face using light downward pressure and lifting the mandible up toward the mask.
   - Reposition the head.
   - Check for secretions; suction mouth and nose.
   - Ventilate with the baby's mouth slightly open.
   - Increase pressure of ventilations.
   - Recheck or replace the resuscitation bag.
   - After reasonable attempts fail, intubate the baby.

10. Improvement during positive-pressure ventilation with a mask is indicated by a rapid increase in heart rate and subsequent improvement in
    - Color and oxygen saturation
    - Muscle tone
    - Spontaneous breathing

Key Points — *continued*

11. Current evidence is insufficient to resolve all questions regarding supplemental oxygen use for positive-pressure ventilation during neonatal resuscitation.

    • The Neonatal Resuscitation Program recommends use of 100% supplemental oxygen when positive-pressure ventilation is required during neonatal resuscitation.

    • However, research suggests that resuscitation with something less than 100% may be just as successful.

    • If resuscitation is started with room air, supplemental oxygen, up to 100%, should be administered if there is no appreciable improvement within 90 seconds following birth.

    • If supplemental oxygen is unavailable, use room air to deliver positive-pressure ventilation.

Lesson 3 Review

(The answers follow.)

1. Flow-inflating bags (will) (will not) work without a compressed gas source.

2. A baby is born apneic and cyanotic. You clear his airway and stimulate him. Thirty seconds after birth, he has not improved. The next step is to (stimulate him more) (begin positive-pressure ventilation).

3. The single most important and most effective step in neonatal resuscitation is (stimulation) (ventilating the lungs).

4. Label these bags "flow-inflating," "self-inflating," or "T-piece resuscitator."

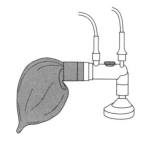

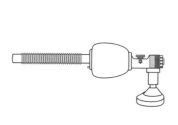

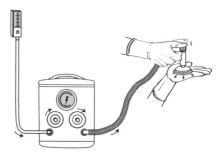

A. _____   B. _____   C. _____

5. Masks of different sizes (do) (do not) need to be available at every delivery.

6. Self-inflating bags require the attachment of a(n) _____ to deliver 90% to 100% oxygen.

7. T-piece resuscitators (will) (will not) work without a compressed gas source.

8. Neonatal ventilation bags are (much smaller than) (the same size as) adult ventilation bags.

9. List the principal safety feature for each of the following devices:

   Self-inflating bag: _____

   Flow-inflating bag: _____

   T-piece resuscitator: _____

10. Free-flow oxygen can be delivered reliably through the mask attached to a (flow-inflating bag) (self-inflating bag) (T-piece resuscitator).

Lesson 3 Review — *continued*

11. When giving free-flow oxygen with a flow-inflating bag and mask, it is necessary to place the mask (securely) (loosely) on the baby's face to allow some gas to escape around the edges of the mask.

12. Which mask is correct?

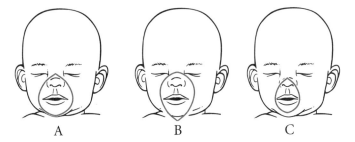

        A   B   C

13. Before an anticipated resuscitation, the ventilation device should be connected to a(n)

_____.

14. Which baby is positioned properly for positive-pressure ventilation?

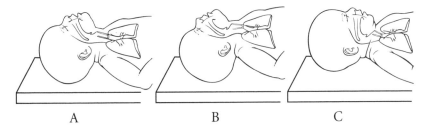

        A   B   C

15. Which illustration(s) shows the correct position for assisting positive-pressure ventilation?

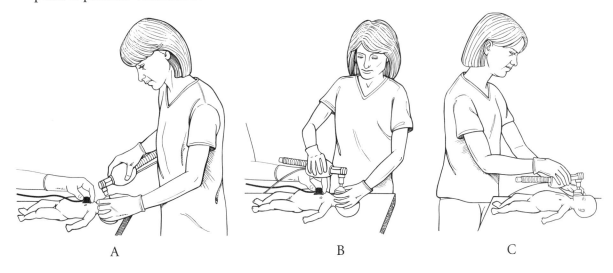

        A   B   C

16. You must hold the resuscitation device so that you can see the newborn's _____ and

_____.

Lesson 3 Review — *continued*

17. An anatomically shaped mask should be positioned with the (pointed) (rounded) end over the newborn's nose.

18. If you notice that the baby's chest looks as if he is taking deep breaths, you are (overinflating) (underinflating) the lungs, and it is possible that a pneumothorax may occur.

19. When ventilating a baby, you should provide positive-pressure ventilation at a rate of _____ to _____ breaths per minute.

20. Before stopping assisted ventilation, you should note improvement in the following 4 physical signs:

    (1)_____

    (2)_____

    (3)_____

    (4)_____

21. You are using a self-inflating bag to ventilate a baby. The bag fills after every squeeze. The baby's heart rate, color, and muscle tone are not improving and there is no perceptible chest movement with each breath. List 3 possibilities of what may be wrong.

    (1)_____

    (2)_____

    (3)_____

22. If, after making appropriate adjustments, you are unable to obtain physiologic improvement and chest expansion with positive-pressure ventilation, you usually will have to insert a(n) _____.

23. You notice that a baby's heart rate, color, and muscle tone are improving and the baby's chest is moving as you provide positive-pressure ventilation. Another way to check for good aeration is to use a _____ to listen for _____ sounds in both lungs.

24. If you must continue positive-pressure ventilation with a mask for more than several minutes, a(n) _____ should be inserted to act as a vent for the gas in the stomach during the remainder of the resuscitation.

Lesson 3 Review — *continued*

25. How far should this orogastric catheter be inserted? _____ cm

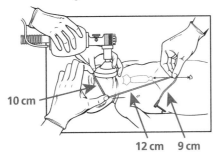

26. As soon as the orogastric catheter is inserted, a syringe is attached and gastric contents are removed. Then the syringe is removed, and the catheter is left _____ to vent stomach gas.

27. The vast majority of babies requiring resuscitation (will) (will not) improve with positive-pressure ventilation.

Lesson 3 Answers to Questions

1. Flow-inflating bags **will not** work without a compressed gas source.

2. The next step is to **begin positive-pressure ventilation.**

3. **Ventilating the lungs** is the most important and effective step in neonatal resuscitation.

4. A. **flow-inflating;** B. **self-inflating;** C. **T-piece resuscitator**

5. Masks of different sizes **do** need to be at every delivery.

6. Self-inflating bags require the attachment of an **oxygen reservoir** to deliver 90% to 100% oxygen.

7. T-piece resuscitators **will not** work without a compressed gas source.

8. Neonatal ventilation bags are **much smaller than** adult ventilation bags.

9. Self-inflating bag: **Pop-off valve and optional pressure gauge**
   Flow-inflating bag: **Pressure gauge**
   T-piece resuscitator: **Maximum pressure relief control and pressure gauge**

10. Free-flow oxygen can be delivered reliably with a **flow-inflating bag and T-piece resuscitator,** but not through the mask of a self-inflating bag.

11. When giving free-flow oxygen, place the mask **loosely** on the baby's face to allow some gas to escape around the edges of the mask.

12. Mask **A** is correct.

13. The device should be connected to **an oxygen source.**

14. Baby **A** is positioned correctly.

15. Illustrations **A and B** are correct.

16. You should be able to see the newborn's **chest** and **abdomen.**

17. An anatomically shaped mask should be positioned with the **pointed** end over the newborn's nose.

Answers to Questions — *continued*

18. You are **overinflating** the lungs, and there is danger you will produce a pneumothorax.

19. Squeeze the resuscitation bag at a rate of **40** to **60** breaths per minute.

20. You should note improvement in (1) **heart rate,** (2) **color,** (3) **breathing,** and (4) **improving muscle tone.**

21. If the heart rate, color, and muscle tone are not improving and the chest is not moving, there may be (1) **an inadequate seal between the mask and face,** (2) **a blocked airway,** or (3) **insufficient pressure.**

22. You usually will have to insert an **endotracheal tube.**

23. Use a **stethoscope** to listen for **breath** sounds in both lungs.

24. An **orogastric tube** should be inserted to act as a vent for the gas in the stomach.

25. The orogastric catheter should be inserted **22** cm (10 cm + 12 cm).

26. The syringe is removed, and the catheter is left **open** to vent stomach gas.

27. The vast majority of babies requiring resuscitation **will** improve with positive-pressure ventilation.

Performance Checklist

Lesson 3 — Positive-Pressure Ventilation

Instructor: The learner should be instructed to talk through the procedure as it is demonstrated. Judge the performance of each step and check (✓) the box when the action is completed correctly. If done incorrectly, circle the box so that you can discuss that step later. You will need to provide information at several points concerning the condition of the baby. If the institution policy is that a T-piece resuscitator normally is used in the delivery room, the learner should demonstrate proficiency with that device. However, he or she also should demonstrate ability to use a bag and mask.

Learner: To successfully complete this checklist, you should be able to perform all the steps and make all the correct decisions in the procedure. You should talk through the procedure as you perform it.

> **Equipment and Supplies**
>
> Newborn resuscitation manikin
>
> Radiant warmer or table to simulate warmer
>
> Gloves (or may simulate this)
>
> Bulb syringe or suction catheter
>
> Stethoscope
>
> Shoulder roll
>
> Self-inflating bag
> - With positive end-expiratory pressure valve (optional)
>
> or
>
> Flow-inflating bag with pressure gauge and oxygen source
>
> and (if this device is used in the delivery room)
>
> T-piece resuscitator and components
>
> Flowmeter (or may simulate this)
>
> Oxygen/air blender (optional)
>
> Masks (term and preterm sizes)
>
> Method to administer free-flow oxygen (oxygen mask, oxygen tubing, flow-inflating bag and mask, or T-piece resuscitator)
>
> Feeding tube and syringe
>
> Tape
>
> Clock with second hand

Birth

Approximate Time

30 sec
- **Term gestation?**
- **Clear amniotic fluid?**
- **Breathing or crying?**
- **Good muscle tone?**

No

- **Provide warmth**
- **Position; clear airway*** **(as necessary)**
- **Dry, stimulate, reposition**

- **Evaluate respirations, heart rate, and color**

Breathing, HR >100 but cyanotic

Apneic or HR <100

- **Give supplemental oxygen**

Persistently cyanotic

30 sec

- **Provide positive-pressure ventilation***

Effective ventilation **HR >100 & Pink**

Post-resuscitation Care

*** Endotracheal intubation may be considered at several steps.**

Performance Checklist

Lesson 3 — Positive-Pressure Ventilation

Name _____ Instructor _____ Date _____

Instructor's questions are in quotes. Learner's questions and correct responses are in bold type. Instructor should check boxes as the learner answers correctly.

"You are called to the delivery of a baby with an estimated gestation of _____ weeks. How would you prepare the ventilation equipment for this baby? You may ask me anything you would like to know about the baby's condition as you progress."

☐ **Selects resuscitation device and connects to oxygen source capable of delivering 90% to 100% oxygen**

☐ **Selects appropriate-sized mask**

☐ **Tests resuscitation device:**
- **Good pressure?**
- **Pressure release valve working (self-inflating bag)?**
- **Valve assembly present and working (self-inflating bag)?**
- **Flow control valve adjusted (flow-inflating bag)?**
- **Controls set on device (T-piece resuscitator)?**
  - **Maximum circuit pressure**
  - **Peak inspiratory pressure**
  - **Positive end-expiratory pressure**

"The baby has just been born, placed under the radiant warmer, positioned, suctioned, dried, and given tactile stimulation. The baby is still apneic. Demonstrate what you would do for this baby."

☐ **Positions himself or herself at the head or side of the baby and positions baby's head in "sniffing" position**

☐ **Calls for assistance**

☐ **Positions mask properly on baby**

☐ **Begins ventilations at appropriate rate and pressure**

☐ **Asks assistant to report heart rate and breath sounds**

"Heart rate improving" "Heart rate not improving"

☐ **Looks for chest movement; asks about breath sounds**

Chest movement No chest movement

☐ **Checks for inadequate seal and head position**

Corrects seal and position Good seal and position

Performance Checklist — *continued*

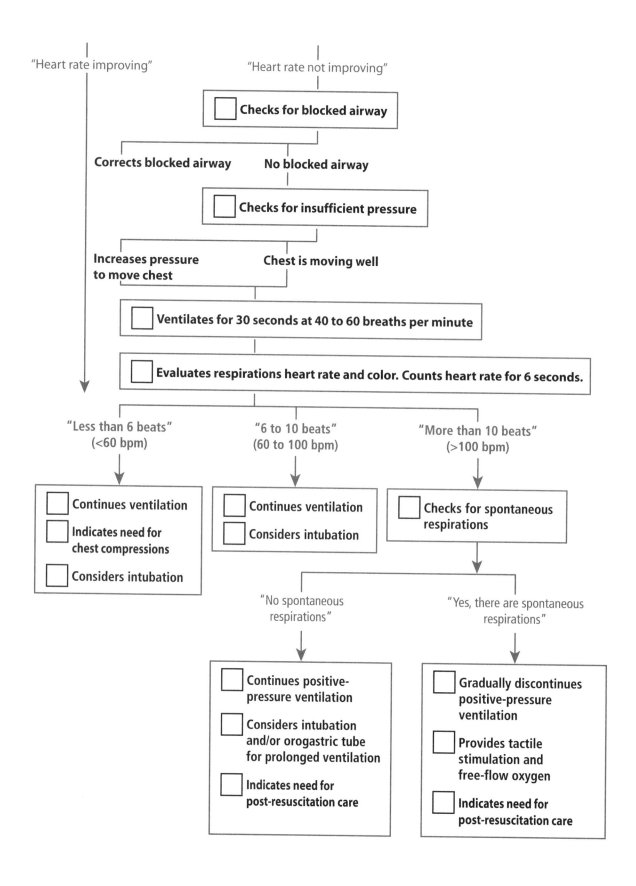

"Heart rate improving"

"Heart rate not improving"

☐ Checks for blocked airway

Corrects blocked airway   No blocked airway

☐ Checks for insufficient pressure

Increases pressure to move chest   Chest is moving well

☐ Ventilates for 30 seconds at 40 to 60 breaths per minute

☐ Evaluates respirations heart rate and color. Counts heart rate for 6 seconds.

"Less than 6 beats" (<60 bpm)

"6 to 10 beats" (60 to 100 bpm)

"More than 10 beats" (>100 bpm)

☐ Continues ventilation

☐ Indicates need for chest compressions

☐ Considers intubation

☐ Continues ventilation

☐ Considers intubation

☐ Checks for spontaneous respirations

"No spontaneous respirations"

"Yes, there are spontaneous respirations"

☐ Continues positive-pressure ventilation

☐ Considers intubation and/or orogastric tube for prolonged ventilation

☐ Indicates need for post-resuscitation care

☐ Gradually discontinues positive-pressure ventilation

☐ Provides tactile stimulation and free-flow oxygen

☐ Indicates need for post-resuscitation care

Performance Checklist — *continued*

Instructor should present each of the scenarios separately and evaluate the learner's response for each.

- [ ] Correctly calculated baby's heart rate from 6-second count.
- [ ] Speed—no undue delays.
- [ ] Handling of baby was safe, with no trauma produced.
- [ ] Ventilated at appropriate rate (40 to 60 breaths per minute).
- [ ] Ventilated with appropriate pressure.
- [ ] Avoided using excessive pressure on mask.
- [ ] If ventilation continued longer than several minutes, an orogastric tube was inserted.

Appendix

Read the section(s) that refers to the type of device used in your hospital.

A. Self-inflating resuscitation bags

What are the parts of a self-inflating bag?

There are 7 basic parts to a self-inflating bag
(Figure 3A.1).

1. Air inlet and attachment site for oxygen
   reservoir
2. Oxygen inlet
3. Patient outlet
4. Valve assembly
5. Oxygen reservoir
6. Pressure-release (pop-off) valve
7. Pressure gauge or pressure gauge
   attachment site (optional)

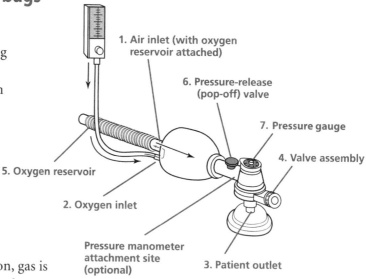

1. Air inlet (with oxygen reservoir attached)
6. Pressure-release (pop-off) valve
7. Pressure gauge
4. Valve assembly
5. Oxygen reservoir
2. Oxygen inlet
Pressure manometer attachment site (optional)
3. Patient outlet

As the bag re-expands following compression, gas is
drawn into the bag through a one-way valve that may
be located at either end of the bag, depending on the
design. This valve is called the *air inlet.*

Figure 3A.1. Parts of a self-inflating bag

Every self-inflating bag has an *oxygen inlet,* which usually is located
near the air inlet. The oxygen inlet is a small nipple or projection to
which oxygen tubing is attached. In the self-inflating bag, an oxygen
tube does not need to be attached for the bag to function. The oxygen
tube should be attached when the bag is to be used for neonatal
resuscitation.

The *patient outlet* is where gas exits from the bag to the baby and
where the mask or endotracheal tube attaches.

Most self-inflating bags have a *pressure-release valve* that prevents
excessive pressure buildup in the bag. Some self-inflating bags have a
pressure gauge or site for attaching a pressure gauge. The attachment
site usually consists of a small hole or projection close to the patient
outlet. If your bag has such a site, either the hole must be plugged or
the gauge must be attached. Otherwise, gas will leak through the
opening, preventing adequate pressure from being generated. Care
should be taken to avoid connecting the oxygen inflow tubing to the
site for attaching the pressure gauge, if present. High pressure may be
generated in the baby and cause a pneumothorax or other air leak.
Attach the oxygen tubing and pressure transducer according to
manufacturer instructions.

Appendix — *continued*

Self-inflating bags have a *valve assembly* positioned between the bag and the patient outlet (Figure 3A.2). When the bag is squeezed during ventilation, the valve opens, releasing oxygen/air to the patient. When the bag reinflates (during the exhalation phase of the cycle), the valve is closed. This prevents the patient's exhaled air from entering the bag and being re-breathed. You should become familiar with the valve assembly—what it looks like and how it responds as you squeeze and release the bag. If it is missing or malfunctioning, the bag should not be used.

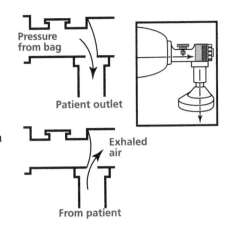

Figure 3A.2. Principle of valve assembly of a self-inflating bag

Why is an oxygen reservoir necessary on a self-inflating bag?

Current recommendations are that most babies who require resuscitation with assisted ventilation at birth should be ventilated initially with supplemental oxygen. The amount of supplemental oxygen during positive-pressure ventilation will be discussed later in this lesson and in Lesson 8.

Oxygen enters a self-inflating bag through tubing connected between an oxygen source and the oxygen inlet port on the bag. However, each time the bag reinflates after you squeeze it, room air, containing 21% oxygen, is drawn into the bag through the air inlet. The air dilutes the concentration of oxygen in the bag. Therefore, even though you may have 100% oxygen flowing through the oxygen inlet, it is diluted by the air that enters each time the bag reinflates. As a result, the concentration of oxygen actually received by the patient is reduced to about 40% (Figure 3A.3). (The actual concentration will depend on the flow rate of oxygen coming from the source and how frequently the bag is squeezed.)

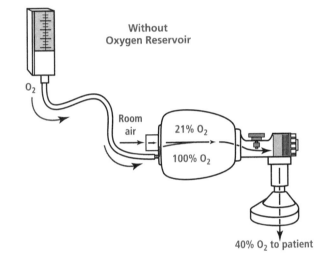

Figure 3A.3. Self-inflating bag without an oxygen reservoir delivers only 40% oxygen to the patient

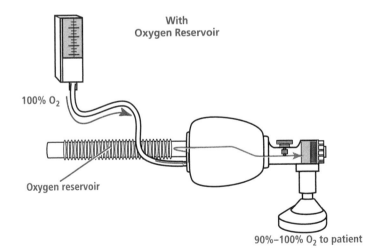

Figure 3A.4. Self-inflating bag with oxygen reservoir delivers 90% to 100% oxygen to the patient

Concentrations of oxygen higher than 40% can be achieved with a self-inflating bag by using an *oxygen reservoir.* An oxygen reservoir is an appliance that can be placed over the bag's air inlet (Figure 3A.4). The reservoir allows 90% to 100% oxygen to collect at the air inlet, thus preventing the oxygen from being diluted with room air. However, the flow of oxygen is delivered reliably to the patient only when the bag is squeezed. When the bag is not being squeezed, a high concentration of oxygen escapes from the open end of the oxygen reservoir.

Appendix — *continued*

Several different types of oxygen reservoirs are available, but they all perform the same function. Some have open ends and others have a valve that allows some air to enter the reservoir (Figure 3A.5). Therefore, the concentration of oxygen achieved with a self-inflating bag with an oxygen reservoir attached will be between 90% and 100%.

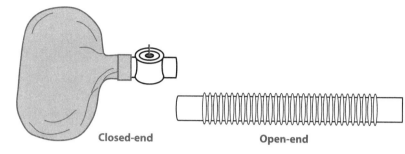

Closed-end   Open-end

Figure 3A.5. Different types of oxygen reservoirs for self-inflating bags

How do you test a self-inflating bag before use?

First, be certain that the oxygen tubing and oxygen reservoir are connected. Adjust the flow to 5 to 10 L/min.

To check the operation of a self-inflating bag, block the mask or patient outlet with the palm of your hand and squeeze the bag (Figure 3A.6).

- Do you feel pressure against your hand?

- Can you force the pressure-release valve open?

- Does the pressure gauge (if present) register 30 to 40 cm H_2O pressure when the pressure release valve opens?

If not,

- Is there a crack or leak in the bag?

- Is the pressure gauge missing, resulting in an open attachment site?

- Is the pressure-release valve missing or stuck closed?

- Is the patient outlet sufficiently blocked?

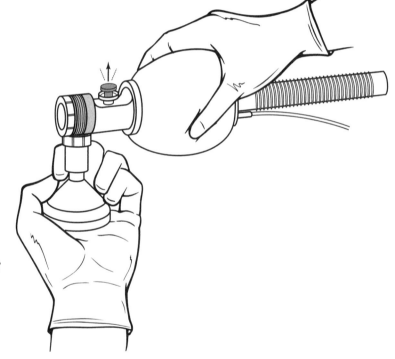

Figure 3A.6. Testing a self-inflating bag

If your bag generates adequate pressure and the safety features are working while the mask-patient outlet is blocked,

- Does the bag reinflate quickly when you release your grip?

If there is any problem with the bag, obtain a new one. Self-inflating bags usually have more parts than flow-inflating bags. During cleaning, parts may be left out or assembled incorrectly. If parts remain moist after cleaning, they may stick together.

Appendix — *continued*

How do you control pressure in a self-inflating bag?

The amount of pressure delivered by a self-inflating bag is not dependent on the flow of oxygen entering the bag. When you seal the mask on the baby's face (or connect the bag to an endotracheal tube), there will be no change in the inflation of a self-inflating bag. The amount of pressure and volume delivered with each breath depends on the following 3 factors:

- How hard you squeeze the bag
- Any leak that may be present between the mask and the baby's face
- The set-point of the pressure-release valve

Review—*Appendix A*

(The answers are in the preceding section and at the end of the Appendix.)

A-1. A self-inflating bag with a pressure gauge site will work only if a pressure gauge is connected to the site or if the connection site is (left open) (plugged).

A-2. A self-inflating bag can deliver 90% to 100% oxygen (by itself) (only when an oxygen reservoir is attached).

A-3. A self-inflating bag connected to 100% oxygen, but without an oxygen reservoir attached to it, delivers only about _____% oxygen.

A-4. You are testing a resuscitation bag. When you squeeze the bag, you (should) (should not) feel pressure against your hand.

A-5. If a pressure gauge was present (see illustration at right), what should it read when you squeeze the bag?

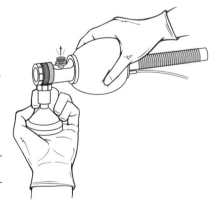

_____

A-6. List 3 important factors that determine the peak inspiratory pressure delivered from a self-inflating bag.

(1)_____

(2)_____

(3)_____

Appendix — *continued*

B. Flow-inflating resuscitation bags

What are the parts of a flow-inflating bag?
There are 4 parts to a flow-inflating bag
(Figure 3B.1).

1. Oxygen inlet

2. Patient outlet

3. Flow-control valve

4. Pressure gauge attachment site

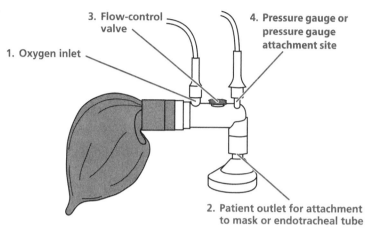

Oxygen from a compressed source (or an
oxygen-air mixture from a blender) enters
the bag at the *oxygen inlet.* The inlet is a
small projection designed to fit oxygen
tubing. The inlet may be at either end of
the device, depending on the brand and model you use.

Figure 3B.1. Parts of a flow-inflating bag

Oxygen (at whatever concentration entered at the inlet) exits from the
bag to the patient at the *patient outlet,* where the mask or
endotracheal tube attaches to the device.

The *flow-control* valve provides an adjustable leak that allows you to
regulate the pressure in the bag when the bag is connected to an
endotracheal tube or the mask is held tightly on the patient's face. The
adjustable opening provides an additional outlet for the incoming gas
and allows excess gas to escape rather than overinflate the bag or be
forced into the patient.

Flow-inflating bags usually have a *site for attaching a pressure gauge*
(Figure 3B.2). The attachment site usually is close to the patient outlet.
The pressure gauge registers the amount of pressure you are using to
ventilate the newborn. If your flow-inflating bag has a connecting site
for a pressure gauge, a gauge must be attached to the site. If the gauge
is absent, the attachment site must be occluded with a plug or the site
will be a source of leak and the bag will not inflate properly.

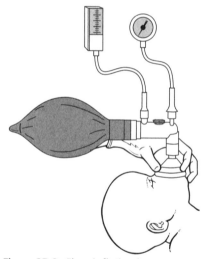

Figure 3B.2. Flow-inflating bag
attached to oxygen source and
pressure manometer

Appendix — *continued*

How does a flow-inflating bag work?

For a flow-inflating bag to work properly, there must be adequate gas flow from the source and a sealed system. The bag will not inflate adequately if (Figure 3B.3)

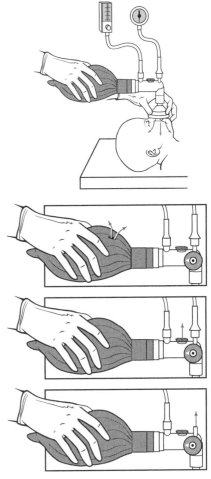

- The mask is not properly sealed against the baby's face.
- The flow from the source is insufficient.

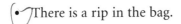 • There is a rip in the bag.

- The flow-control valve is open too far.

- The pressure gauge is not attached or the oxygen tubing has become disconnected or occluded.

Figure 3B.3. Reasons for failure of the flow-inflating bag to inflate

Appendix — *continued*

How do you test a flow-inflating bag before use?

To check a flow-inflating bag, attach it to a gas source. Adjust the flowmeter to 5 to 10 L/min. Block the patient outlet to make sure the bag fills properly (Figure 3B.4). Do this by making a seal between the mask and the palm of your hand. Adjust the flow-control valve so that the bag is not over-distended. Watch the pressure gauge, and adjust the valve so that there is approximately 5 cm H_2O pressure when the bag is not being squeezed, and 30 to 40 cm H_2O peak inflation pressure when the bag is squeezed firmly.

Does the bag fill properly? If not,

- Is there a crack or tear in the bag?
- Is the flow-control valve open too far?
- Is the pressure gauge attached?
- Is the oxygen line connected securely?
- Is the patient outlet sufficiently blocked?

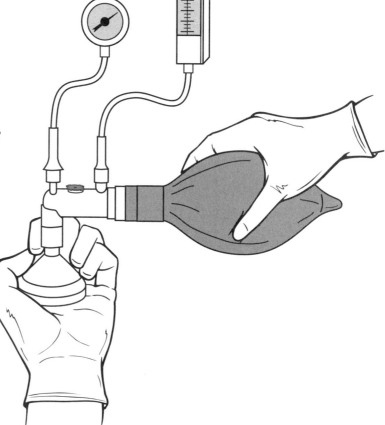

Figure 3B.4. Testing a flow-inflating bag

If the bag fills, squeeze the bag.

- Do you feel pressure against your hand?
- Does the pressure gauge register 5 cm H_2O pressure when not squeezed, and 30 to 40 cm H_2O when squeezed firmly?

Squeeze the bag at a rate of 40 to 60 times per minute and pressures of 40 cm H_2O. If the bag does not fill rapidly enough, readjust the flow-control valve or increase the gas flow from the flowmeter. Then check to be sure that the pressure gauge still reads 5 cm H_2O pressure when the bag is not being squeezed. You may need to make further adjustments in the flow-control valve to avoid excessive end-expiratory pressure.

If the bag still does not fill properly or does not generate adequate pressure, get another bag and begin again.

Appendix — *continued*

How do you adjust the oxygen flow, concentration, and pressure in a flow-inflating bag?

When using a flow-inflating bag, you inflate the bag with compressed gas (oxygen or an oxygen-air mixture from a blender) (Figure 3B.5). The flow should be adjusted to 5 to 10 L/min and may need to be increased if the bag does not fill sufficiently. Once the gas enters the bag, it is not diluted as it is in a self-inflating bag. Therefore, whatever concentration of oxygen that enters the bag is the same concentration delivered to the patient. For most resuscitations, this program will recommend delivering positive pressure with 100% oxygen. However, if you want to use less than 100% oxygen, you will need to connect the tubing from the bag to a mixing device that permits you to mix oxygen with compressed air, either from a wall outlet or from a tank. Further discussion of how and when to adjust oxygen concentration to something less than 100% will be presented in Lesson 8.

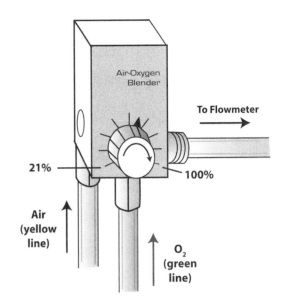

Figure 3B.5. Mixing oxygen and air with an oxygen blender. There is a control knob to dial in the desired oxygen concentration

Once you seal the mask on the baby's face (or connect the bag to an endotracheal tube, as you will learn in Lesson 5), all of the oxygen coming from the wall or blender will be directed to the bag (and thus to the patient), with some coming out the flow-control valve. This will cause the bag to inflate (Figure 3B.6). There are 2 ways that you can adjust the pressure in the bag and thus the amount of inflation of the bag.

- By adjusting the flowmeter, you regulate how much gas enters the bag.

- By adjusting the flow-control valve, you regulate how much gas escapes from the bag.

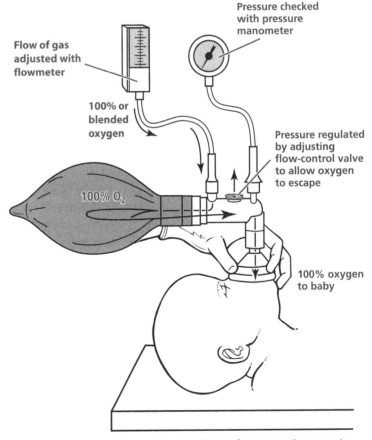

Figure 3B.6. Regulation of oxygen and pressure in flow-inflating bag

Appendix — *continued*

The flowmeter and flow-control valve should be set so that the bag is inflated to the point where it is comfortable to handle and does not completely deflate with each ventilation (Figure 3B.7).

An overinflated bag is difficult to manage and may deliver high pressure to the baby; a pneumothorax or other air leak may develop. An underinflated bag makes it difficult to achieve the desired inflation pressure (Figure 3B.8). With practice, you will be able to make the necessary adjustments to achieve a balance. If there is an adequate seal between the baby's face and the mask, you should be able to maintain the appropriate amount of inflation with the flowmeter set at 5 to 10 L/min.

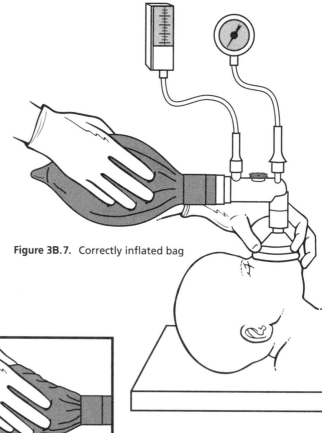

Figure 3B.7. Correctly inflated bag

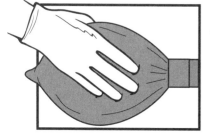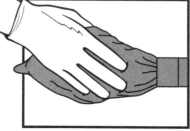

Figure 3B.8. Resuscitation bags that are overinflated (left) and underinflated (right)

Review – *Appendix B*

(The answers are in the preceding section and at the end of the Appendix.)

B-1. List 4 reasons why the flow-inflating bag may fail to ventilate the baby.

(1)_____

(2)_____

(3)_____

(4)_____

B-2. Which flow-inflating bag is being used properly?

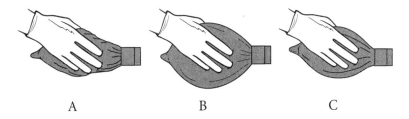

A   B   C

B-3. To regulate the pressure of the oxygen going to the baby with a flow-inflating bag, you may adjust either the flowmeter on the wall or the (flow-control valve) (pressure gauge).

B-4. If the gas flow through the flow-inflating bag is too high, there (is) (is not) an increased risk for pneumothorax.

Appendix — *continued*

C. T-piece Resuscitator

What are the parts of a T-piece resuscitator?

There are 6 parts to a flow-controlled, pressure-limited T-piece resuscitator (Figure 3C.1).

1. Oxygen (gas) inlet
2. Patient (gas) outlet
3. Maximum pressure relief control
4. Circuit pressure gauge
5. Inspiratory pressure control
6. Patient T-piece with positive end-expiratory pressure (PEEP) cap

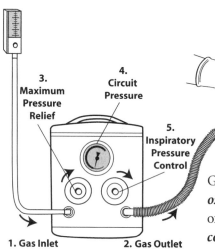

Figure 3C.1. Parts of the T-piece resuscitator

Gas from a compressed source enters the T-piece resuscitator at the *oxygen (gas) inlet.* The inlet is a small projection designed to fit oxygen tubing and is embedded in the *maximum pressure relief control.* The desired maximum pressure is set after occluding the PEEP cap and turning the maximum pressure relief control (see following text) to the maximum pressure limit. The manufacturer of one device has set the default level of 40 cm H_2O; however, this is adjustable.

Oxygen exits from the T-piece resuscitator *patient (gas) outlet* by the *gas supply line* to the *patient T-piece,* where the mask or endotracheal tube attaches.

The *inspiratory pressure control* is used to set the desired peak inspiratory pressure (PIP).

The *PEEP cap* is used to set the positive end-expiratory pressure, if needed.

The *circuit pressure gauge* is used to set and monitor peak inspiratory pressure, positive end-expiratory pressure, and maximum circuit pressure.

How does a T-piece resuscitator work?

The T-piece resuscitator is specially designed for neonatal resuscitation. Pressure controls for maximum circuit pressure, desired PIP, and PEEP must be set by the operator before use (see following text). When the PEEP valve is occluded by the operator, the preset PIP is delivered to the patient for as long as the PEEP valve is occluded.

Appendix — *continued*

How do you prepare the T-piece resuscitator for use?

First, assemble the parts of the T-piece resuscitator as instructed by the manufacturer.

Second, attach a test lung to the patient outlet. The test lung is an inflatable balloon that should have been provided by the device manufacturer.

Third, connect the device to a gas source. This will be a tubing either from a 100% oxygen source or from a blender that permits adjustment of oxygen concentration from 21% to 100%. (See Lesson 2.)

Fourth, adjust the pressure settings as follows:

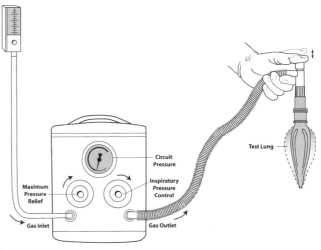

Figure 3C.2. Setting up a T-piece resuscitator

- Adjust the flowmeter to regulate how much gas flows into the T-piece resuscitator (5 to 15 L/min recommended).

- Set the maximum circuit pressure by occluding the PEEP cap with your finger and adjusting the maximum pressure relief dial to a selected value (40 cm H_2O is recommended) (Figure 3C.2).

- Set the desired peak inspiratory pressure by occluding the PEEP cap with your finger and adjusting the inspiratory pressure control to a selected peak inspiratory pressure (Figure 3C.3).

- Set the positive end-expiratory pressure by removing your finger from the PEEP cap and adjusting the PEEP cap to the desired setting (0 to 5 cm H_2O is recommended). (See Lesson 8.)

- Remove the test lung and attach the patient T-piece resuscitator to a face mask or be prepared to attach it to an endotracheal tube after the trachea has been intubated. (See Lesson 5.)

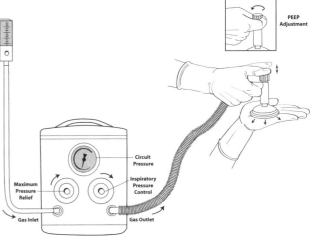

Figure 3C.3. Adjusting the maximum and peak pressure before use

After the device is connected to the patient, either by applying the mask to the patient or by connecting the device to an endotracheal tube, you will control the respiratory rate by intermittently occluding the PEEP cap.

If you want to change the peak inflation pressure, you will need to readjust the inspiratory pressure control. This can be done while you are ventilating the patient and will not require reattaching the test lung.

Appendix — *continued*

How do you adjust the concentration of oxygen in a T-piece resuscitator?

The concentration of oxygen supplying the T-piece resuscitator is the same as that delivered to the baby. Therefore, if the T-piece resuscitator is connected to a source of 100% oxygen, 100% oxygen will be delivered to the baby. To deliver less than 100%, you will have to have a source of compressed air and have the device connected to an oxygen blender. The blender can then be adjusted from 21% to 100%.

What may be wrong if the baby doesn't improve or the desired peak pressure is not reached?

*   The mask may not be properly sealed on the baby's face.
*   The gas supply may not be connected or of sufficient flow.
*   The maximum circuit pressure, peak inspiratory pressure, or end-expiratory pressure may be incorrectly set.

Can you give free-flow oxygen using a T-piece resuscitator?

Free-flow oxygen can be given reliably with a T-piece resuscitator (Figure 3C.4) if you occlude the PEEP cap and hold the mask loosely on the face. The flow rate of oxygen or gas entering the T-piece resuscitator is the same flow rate that exits the patient T-piece toward the baby when the PEEP cap is occluded. When the mask is held loosely on the face, the flow is maintained without generating pressure as the oxygen or gas diffuses into the environment around the mouth and nares.

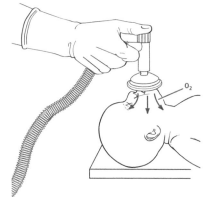

Figure 3C.4. Free-flow oxygen given by a T-piece resuscitator

Review – *Appendix C*

(The answers are in the preceding section and at the end of the Appendix.)

C-1. What pressures must be set before using a T-piece resuscitator?

- _____

- _____

- _____

C-2. The flow rate on a T-piece resuscitator may need to be (increased) (decreased) if the desired peak inspiratory pressure cannot be obtained.

C-3. Free-flow oxygen administered through a T-piece resuscitator requires the PEEP cap to be (open) (occluded).

C-4. T-piece resuscitators (will) (will not) work without a compressed gas source.

Answers to Questions in Appendix

A-1. For a self-inflating bag to work, either the pressure gauge must be connected or the connection site must be **plugged.**

A-2. A self-inflating bag can deliver 90% to 100% oxygen **only when an oxygen reservoir is attached to it.**

A-3. Without an oxygen reservoir, a self-inflating bag can deliver only about **40%** oxygen.

A-4. When you squeeze the bag, you **should** feel pressure against your hand.

A-5. The pressure gauge should read **30 to 40 cm H_2O.**

A-6. The pressure delivered from a self-inflating bag is determined by (1) **how hard you squeeze the bag,** (2) **any leak that may be present between the mask and the baby's face,** and (3) **the set-point of the pressure-release valve.**

B-1. The flow-inflating bag may fail to ventilate the baby because of (1) **an inadequate seal between the mask and the face,** (2) **a tear in the bag,** (3) **the flow-control valve is open too far,** and/or (4) **the pressure gauge is not attached or the oxygen tubing is disconnected or occluded.**

B-2. Illustration **C** is correct.

B-3. Pressure may be regulated by adjusting either the flowmeter or the **flow-control valve.**

B-4. If the gas flow through the flow-inflating bag is too high, there **is** an increased risk for pneumothorax.

C-1. The pressures set on a T-piece resuscitator are

    A. Maximum circuit pressure

    B. Peak inspiratory pressure

    C. Positive end-expiratory pressure

C-2. The flow set on a T-piece resuscitator may need to be **increased** if the desired peak inspiratory pressure cannot be obtained.

C-3. Free-flow oxygen administered through a T-piece resuscitator requires the PEEP cap to be **occluded.**

C-4. T-piece resuscitators **will not** work without a compressed gas source.

4

Chest Compressions

In Lesson 4 you will learn

- When to begin chest compressions during a resuscitation
- How to administer chest compressions
- How to coordinate chest compressions with positive-pressure ventilation
- When to stop chest compressions

The following case is an example of how chest compressions are delivered during a more extensive resuscitation. As you read the case, imagine yourself as part of the resuscitation team. The details of this step will be described in the remainder of the lesson.

Case 4.
Resuscitation with positive-pressure ventilation and chest compressions

A pregnant woman contacts her obstetrician after noticing a pronounced decrease in fetal movements at 34 weeks' gestation.

She is admitted to the labor and delivery unit where persistent fetal bradycardia is noted. Additional skilled personnel are called to the delivery room, the radiant warmer is turned on, and resuscitation equipment is prepared. An emergency cesarean section is performed, and a limp, apneic baby is transferred to the neonatal team.

The team positions the baby's head, suctions his mouth and nose, stimulates him with drying and flicking the soles of his feet, and removes the wet linen. However, 30 seconds after birth, the baby is still limp, cyanotic, and without spontaneous respirations.

One member of the team begins positive-pressure ventilation with a bag and mask using supplemental oxygen, while a second member feels the umbilical cord for the pulse and listens with a stethoscope for breath sounds. The heart rate remains below 60 beats per minute (bpm), despite the presence of breath sounds, and a gentle rise and fall of the chest is noted. After 30 seconds of this, the baby has a very low heart rate (20 to 30 bpm) and remains cyanotic and limp.

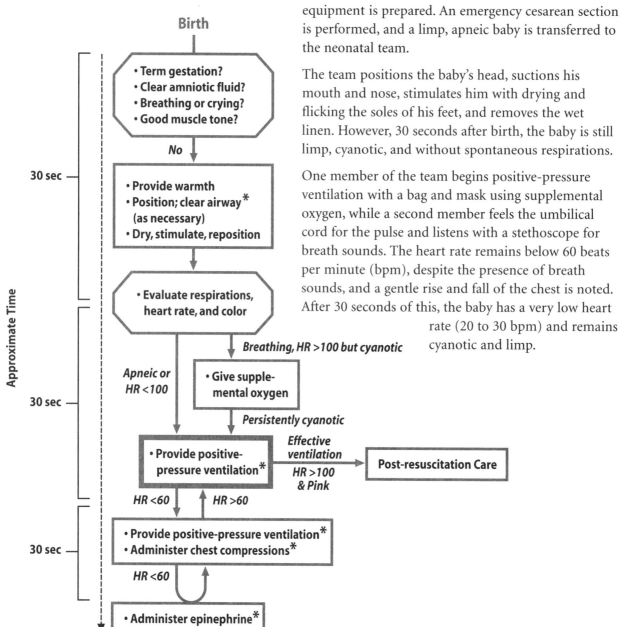

* Endotracheal intubation may be considered at several steps.

The team begins chest compressions coordinated with positive-pressure ventilation. Repeated assessments are made to be certain that the airway is clear and the head is positioned correctly. However, after another 30 seconds, ventilation with the bag and mask does not result in an increased heart rate and ventilation is now not adequately moving the chest.

The trachea is rapidly intubated to ensure effective ventilation, and coordinated chest compressions and positive-pressure ventilation are resumed. Positive-pressure ventilation now results in an increasing heart rate and seems to be producing better chest movement.

The baby finally makes an initial gasp. Chest compressions are stopped when the heart rate rises above 60 bpm. The team continues assisted ventilation. His color improves, and the heart rate rises to more than 100 bpm. After he shows some spontaneous respirations, he is moved to the nursery for careful monitoring and further management.

What are the indications for beginning chest compressions?

Chest compressions are indicated whenever the heart rate remains less than 60 bpm, despite 30 seconds of *effective* positive-pressure ventilation.

Why perform chest compressions?

Babies who have a heart rate below 60 bpm, despite stimulation and 30 seconds of positive-pressure ventilation, probably have very low blood oxygen levels and significant acidosis. As a result, the myocardium is depressed and unable to contract strongly enough to pump blood to the lungs to pick up the oxygen that you have now ensured is in the lungs. Therefore, you will need to mechanically pump blood through the heart while you simultaneously continue to ventilate the lungs until the myocardium becomes sufficiently oxygenated to recover adequate spontaneous function. This process also will help restore oxygen delivery to the brain.

Endotracheal intubation at this time may help ensure adequate ventilation and facilitate the coordination of ventilation and chest compressions.

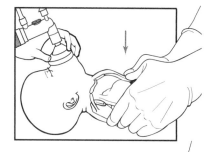

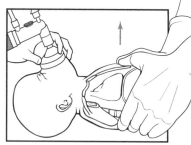

Figure 4.1. Compression (top) and release (bottom) phases of chest compressions

What are chest compressions?

Chest compressions, sometimes referred to as *cardiac massage*, consist of rhythmic compressions of the sternum that

· Compress the heart against the spine.

· Increase the intrathoracic pressure.

· Circulate blood to the vital organs of the body.

The heart lies in the chest between the lower third of the sternum and the spine. Compressing the sternum compresses the heart and increases the pressure in the chest, causing blood to be pumped into the arteries (Figure 4.1).

When pressure on the sternum is released, blood enters the heart from the veins.

How many people are needed to administer chest compressions, and where should they stand?

Remember that chest compressions are of little value unless the lungs are also being ventilated with oxygen. Therefore, 2 people are required to administer effective chest compressions—one to compress the chest and one to continue ventilation. This second person may be the same person who came to monitor heart rate and breath sounds during positive-pressure ventilation.

As you will learn, these 2 people will need to coordinate their activities, so it will be helpful if both of them practice beforehand. The person performing chest compressions must have access to the chest and be able to position his or her hands correctly. The person assisting ventilation will need to be positioned at the baby's head to achieve an effective mask-face seal (or to stabilize the endotracheal tube) and watch for effective chest movement (Figure 4.2).

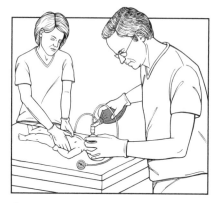

Figure 4.2. Two people are required when chest compressions are given

Neonatal Resuscitation

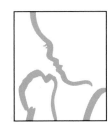

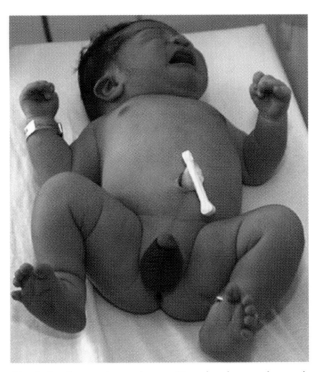

Fig A-1. Normal newborn. Good color and good tone are present. Note absence of central cyanosis and presence of pink color of mucous membranes. Supplemental oxygen is not needed.

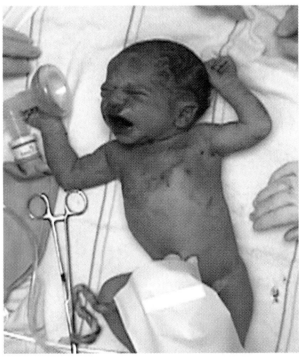

Fig A-2. Cyanosis. This baby has central cyanosis. Supplemental oxygen and perhaps assisted ventilation are needed.

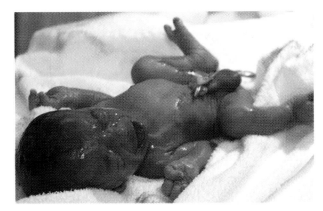

Fig A-3. Newborn immediately following birth. Drying and removing the wet linen will probably stimulate breathing and prevent body cooling.

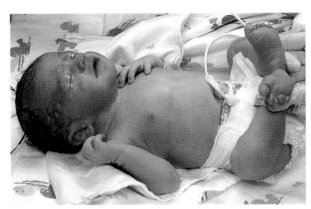

Fig A-4. Acrocyanosis. This baby has acrocyanosis of hands and feet, but trunk and mucous membranes are pink. Supplemental oxygen is not required.

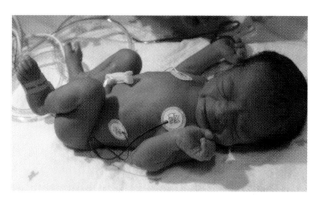

Fig. B-1. At-risk newborn: good tone. This baby is slightly preterm and small for gestational age. However, tone is excellent.

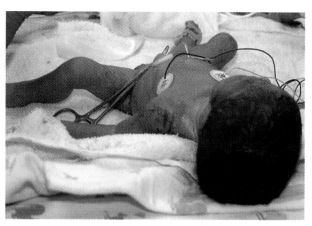

Fig. B-2. At-risk newborn: poor tone. This baby's poor tone is worse than one would anticipate simply from her being born preterm. Resuscitation is required.

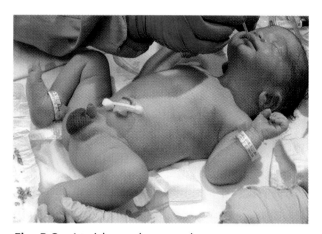

Fig. B-3. At-risk newborn: pale. This baby is very pale and there was a history of placenta previa. Volume expansion may be required.

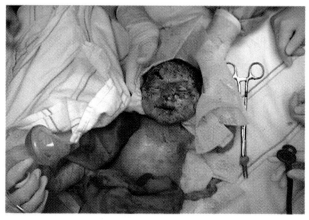

Fig. B-4. At-risk newborn: meconium. This newborn is covered with meconium and is not vigorous (poor tone and poor respiratory effort). Endotracheal intubation and suctioning are required.

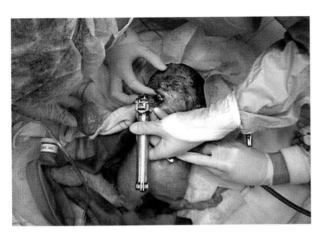

Fig C-1a. Limp baby covered with meconium. Resuscitator is preparing to perform endotracheal intubation and suctioning.

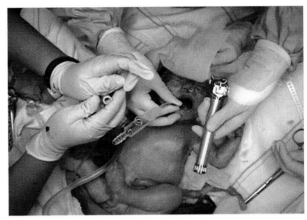

Fig. C-1b. An endotracheal tube has been inserted, a meconium aspiration device has been connected to the tube, and the suction tubing is about to be connected.

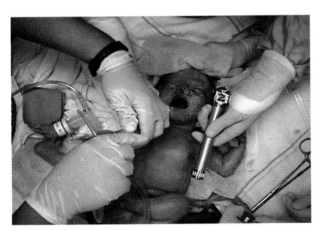

Fig. C-1c. The suction control port is occluded so that the suction is applied to the endotracheal tube as the tube is gradually withdrawn.

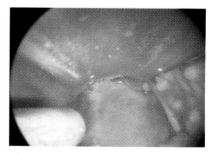

Fig. C-2a. View of posterior pharynx after first inserting laryngoscope.

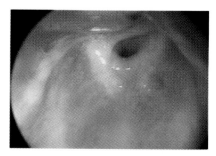

Fig. C-2b. View of esophagus after laryngoscope has been inserted slightly too far.

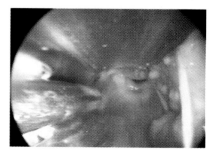

Fig. C-2c. View of arytenoids and posterior glottis as laryngoscope blade is withdrawn slightly.

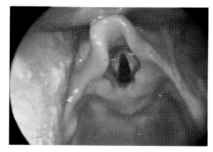

Fig. C-2d. View of glottis and vocal cords as laryngoscope is gently lifted.

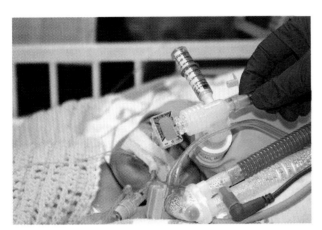

Fig D-1. Violet color of CO_2 detector before being connected to endotracheal tube, thus showing absence of CO_2.

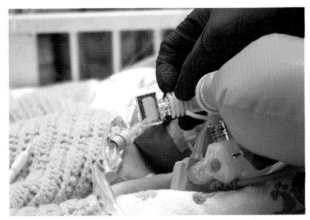

Fig. D-2. Yellow color of CO_2 detector, indicating presence of CO_2 and, therefore, placement of tube within the trachea.

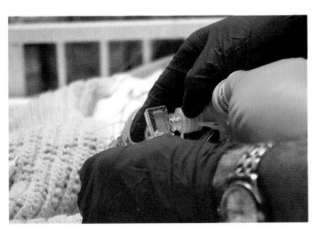

Fig. D-3. Note persistent violet color of CO_2 detector, thus strongly suggesting that the endotracheal tube is in the esophagus, rather than correctly placed in the trachea.

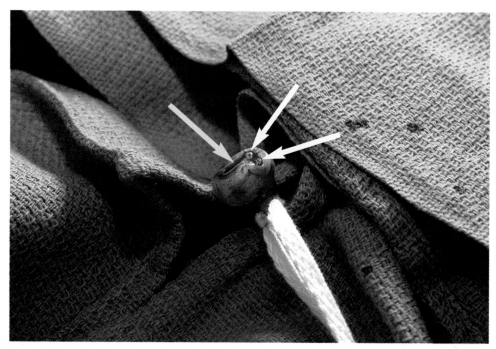

Fig E-1. Cut umbilical cord, before placement of catheter. Note the umbilical arteries (shown by the white arrows) and the umbilical vein (shown by the yellow arrow).

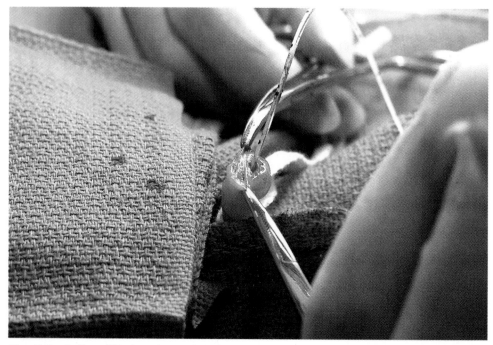

Fig. E-2. Saline-filled catheter has been placed 2 to 4 cm into the umbilical vein (note black centimeter marks on the catheter). Medications should not be administered until blood can be easily aspirated from the catheter.

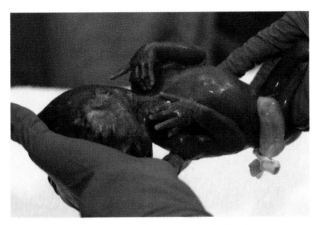

Fig. F-1. This extremely preterm baby is cyanotic, has poor muscle tone, and requires assisted ventilation.

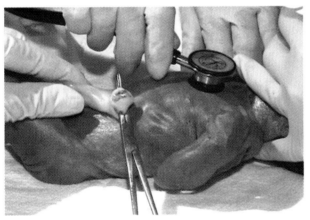

Fig. F-2. Heart rate is being determined by two methods: palpating the base of the cord and listening to the chest.

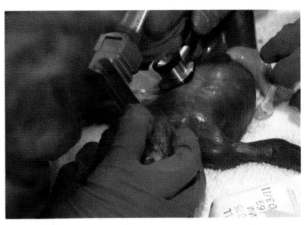

Fig. F-3. Endotracheal intubation procedure is begun as assistant listens to the heart rate.

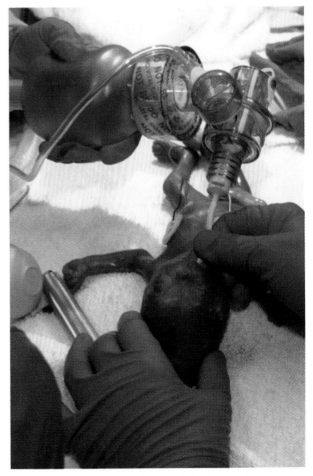

Fig. F-4. Endotracheal tube is held in place as positive-pressure ventilation is provided.

How do you position your hands on the chest to begin chest compressions?

You will learn 2 different techniques for performing chest compressions. These techniques are

- *Thumb technique,* where the 2 thumbs are used to depress the sternum, while the hands encircle the torso and the fingers support the spine (Figure 4.3A).

- *2-finger technique,* where the tips of the middle finger and either the index finger or ring finger of one hand are used to compress the sternum, while the other hand is used to support the baby's back (unless the baby is on a very firm surface) (Figure 4.3B).

What are the advantages of one technique over the other?

Each technique has advantages and disadvantages. Based on a limited amount of data, the thumb technique is preferred, but the 2-finger technique is acceptable.

The thumb technique is preferred because it usually is less tiring, and you can generally control the depth of compression somewhat better. This technique also may be superior in generating peak systolic and coronary perfusion pressure. It also is preferable for individuals with long fingernails. However, the 2-finger technique is more convenient if the baby is large or your hands are small. The 2-finger technique also is preferable to provide access to the umbilicus when medications need to be given by the umbilical route. Therefore, you should learn both techniques.

The 2 techniques have the following things in common:

- Position of the baby

  - Firm support for the back

  - Neck slightly extended

- Compressions

  - Same location, depth, and rate

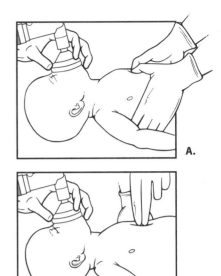

A.

B.

Figure 4.3. Two techniques for giving chest compressions: thumb (A) and 2-finger (B)

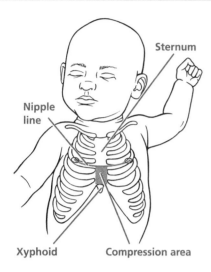

Figure 4.4. Landmarks for chest compressions

Where on the chest should you position your thumbs or fingers?

When chest compressions are performed on a newborn, pressure is applied to the lower third of the sternum, which lies between the xyphoid and a line drawn between the nipples (Figure 4.4). The xyphoid is the small projection where the lower ribs meet at the midline. You can quickly locate the correct area on the sternum by running your fingers along the lower edge of the rib cage until you locate the xyphoid. Then place your thumbs or fingers immediately above the xyphoid. Care must be used to avoid putting pressure directly on the xyphoid.

How do you position your hands using the thumb technique?

The thumb technique is accomplished by encircling the torso with both hands. The thumbs are placed on the sternum and the fingers are under the baby's back, supporting the spine (Figure 4.5).

The thumbs can be placed side by side or, on a small baby, one over the other (Figure 4.5).

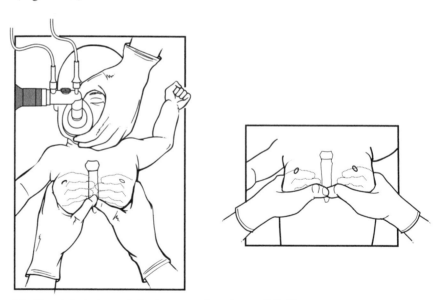

Figure 4.5. Thumb technique of chest compressions for small (left) and large (right) babies

The thumbs will be used to compress the sternum, while your fingers provide the support needed for the back. The thumbs should be flexed at the first joint and pressure applied vertically to compress the heart between the sternum and the spine (Figure 4.6).

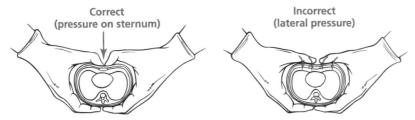

Figure 4.6. Correct and incorrect application of pressure with thumb technique of chest compressions

The thumb technique has some potential disadvantages. It cannot be used effectively if the baby is large or your hands are small. The required position of the rescuer's body also makes access to the umbilical cord somewhat more difficult when medications become necessary.

How do you position your hands using the 2-finger technique?

In the 2-finger technique, the tips of your middle finger and either the index or ring finger of one hand are used for compressions (Figure 4.7). You probably will find it easier to use your right hand if you are right-handed, your left hand if you are left-handed. Position the 2 fingers perpendicular to the chest as shown, and press with your fingertips. If you find that your nails prevent you from using your fingertips, you should ventilate the newborn while your partner compresses the chest. Alternatively, you could use the thumb technique for performing chest compressions.

Your other hand is used to support the newborn's back so that the heart is more effectively compressed between the sternum and spine. With the second hand supporting the back, you can more easily judge the pressure and the depth of compressions.

When compressing the chest, only the 2 fingertips should rest on the chest. This way, you can best control the pressure you apply to the sternum and the spine (Figure 4.8A).

As with the thumb technique, you should apply pressure vertically to compress the heart between the sternum and the spine (Figure 4.8A).

You may find the 2-finger technique to be more tiring than the thumb technique if chest compressions are required for a prolonged period. However, the 2-finger technique can be used regardless of the size of the baby or the size of your hands. An additional advantage of this technique is that it leaves the umbilicus more accessible in case medications must be administered via the umbilical route.

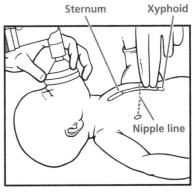

Figure 4.7. Correct finger position for chest compressions

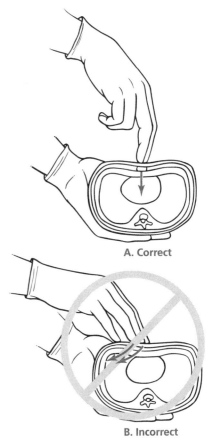

A. Correct

B. Incorrect

Figure 4.8. Correct and incorrect application of pressure with 2-finger technique

Review

(The answers are in the preceding section and at the end of the lesson.)

1. A newborn is apneic and blue. Her airway is cleared, and she is stimulated. At 30 seconds, positive-pressure ventilation is begun. At 60 seconds, her heart rate is 80 beats per minute. Chest compressions (should) (should not) be started. Positive-pressure ventilation (should) (should not) continue.

2. A newborn is apneic and blue. She remains apneic, despite having her airway cleared, being stimulated, and receiving 30 seconds of positive-pressure ventilation. At 60 seconds, her heart rate is 40 beats per minute. Chest compressions (should) (should not) be started. Positive-pressure ventilation (should) (should not) continue.

3. During the compression phase of chest compressions, the sternum compresses the heart, which causes blood to be pumped from the heart into the (veins) (arteries). In the release phase, blood enters the heart from the (veins) (arteries).

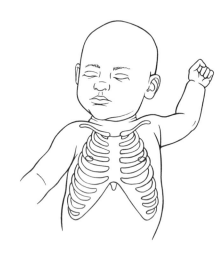

4. Mark the area on this baby (see illustration at left) where you would apply chest compressions.

5. The preferred method of delivering chest compressions is the (thumb) (2-finger) technique.

6. If you anticipate that the baby will need medication by the umbilical route, it may be easier to deliver chest compressions with the (thumb) (2-finger) technique.

How much pressure do you use to compress the chest?

Controlling the pressure used in compressing the sternum is an important part of the procedure.

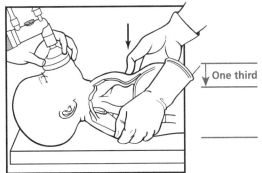

Figure 4.9. Compression depth should be approximately one third of the anterior-posterior diameter of the chest

With your fingers and hands correctly positioned, use enough pressure to depress the sternum *to a depth of approximately one third of the anterior-posterior diameter of the chest* (Figure 4.9), and then release the pressure to allow the heart to refill. One compression consists of the downward stroke plus the release. The actual distance compressed will depend on the size of the baby.

The duration of the downward stroke of the compression also should be somewhat shorter than the duration of the release for generation of maximum cardiac output.

Your thumbs or the tips of your fingers (depending on the method you use) should remain in contact with the chest at all times during both compression *and* release (Figure 4.10). Allow the chest to fully expand by lifting your thumbs or fingers during the release phase to permit blood to reenter the heart from the veins. However, *do not* lift your thumbs or fingers off the chest between compressions (Figure 4.11). If you take your thumbs or fingers completely off the sternum after compression, then

- You waste time relocating the compression area.
- You lose control over the depth of compression.
- You may compress the wrong area, producing trauma to the chest or underlying organs.

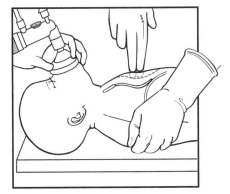

Figure 4.10. *Correct* method of chest compressions (fingers remain in contact with chest on release)

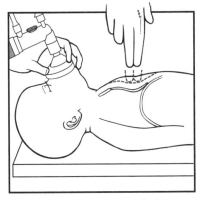

Figure 4.11. *Incorrect* method of chest compressions (fingers lose contact with chest on release)

Are there dangers associated with administering chest compressions?

Chest compressions can cause trauma to the baby.

Two vital organs lie within the rib cage—the heart and lungs. The liver lies partially under the ribs, although it is in the abdominal cavity. As you perform chest compressions, you must apply enough pressure to compress the heart between the sternum and spine without damaging underlying organs. Pressure applied too low, over the xyphoid, can cause laceration of the liver (Figure 4.12).

Also, the ribs are fragile and can be broken easily.

By following the procedure outlined in this lesson, the risk of these injuries can be minimized.

Heart
Lungs
Xyphoid
Liver

Broken ribs

Figure 4.12. Structures that may be damaged during chest compressions

How often do you compress the chest and how do you coordinate compressions with ventilation?

During cardiopulmonary resuscitation, chest compressions must always be accompanied by positive-pressure ventilation. Avoid giving a compression and a ventilation simultaneously, because one will decrease the efficacy of the other. Therefore, the 2 activities must be coordinated, with one ventilation interposed after every third compression, for a total of 30 breaths and 90 compressions per minute (Figure 4.13).

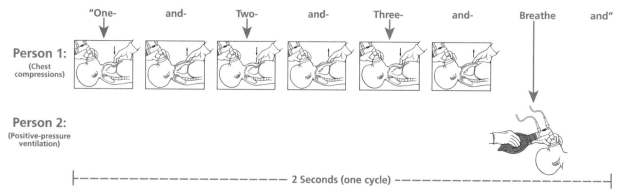

"One-   and-   Two-   and-   Three-   and-   Breathe   and"

Person 1:
(Chest compressions)

Person 2:
(Positive-pressure ventilation)

|———————————— 2 Seconds (one cycle) ————————————|

Figure 4.13. Coordination of chest compressions and ventilation

The person doing the compressions takes over the counting out loud from the person who is doing the ventilating. The compressor counts "One-and-Two-and-Three-and-Breathe-and" while the person ventilating squeezes during "Breathe-and" and releases during "One-and." Note that exhalation occurs during the downward stroke of the next compression. Counting the cadence will help develop a smooth and well-coordinated procedure.

One *cycle of events* will consist of 3 compressions plus 1 ventilation.

• There should be approximately 120 "events" per 60 seconds (1 minute)—90 compressions plus 30 breaths.

Note that, during chest compressions, the ventilation rate is act[u]
30 breaths per minute rather than the rate you previously learn[ed]
positive-pressure ventilation, which was 40 to 60 breaths per mi[nute]
This lower ventilatory rate is needed to provide an adequate nu[mber]
compressions and avoid simultaneous compressions and ventila[tion]
ensure that the process can be coordinated, it is important to p[ractice]
with another person and to practice the roles of both the comp[ressor]
and the ventilator.

How can you practice the rhythm of chest compressions with ventilation?

Imagine that you are the person giving chest compressions. Repeat the words several times while you move your hand to compress the chest on "One-and," "Two-and," "Three-and." Do not press when you say, "Breathe-and." Do not remove your fingers from the surface you are pressing, but be sure to relax your pressure on the chest to permit adequate ventilation during the breath.

Now time yourself to see if you can say and do these 5 cycles of events in 10 seconds. Remember not to press on the "Breathe-and."

Practice saying the words and compressing the chest.

One-and-Two-and-Three-and-Breathe-and-*One-and-Two-and-Three-and*-Breathe-and-

One-and-Two-and-Three-and-Breathe-and-*One-and-Two-and-Three-and*-Breathe-and-

One-and-Two-and-Three-and-Breathe-and

Now imagine that you are the person administering bag-and-mask ventilation. This time you want to squeeze your hand when you say "Breathe-and" but not when you say "One-and," "Two-and," "Three-and."

Now time yourself to see if you can say and do these 5 events in 10 seconds. Remember, squeeze your hand only when you say "Breathe-and."

One-and-Two-and-Three-and-*Breathe-and*-One-and-Two-and-Three-and-*Breathe-and-*

One-and-Two-and-Three-and-*Breathe-and*-One-and-Two-and-Three-and-*Breathe-and-*

One-and-Two-and-Three-and-*Breathe-and*

In a real situation, there will be 2 rescuers, with one doing the compressions and one doing the bagging. The person compressing will be speaking "One-and-Two-and- ..." out loud. Therefore, it is helpful to practice with a partner, taking turns in each of the roles.

When do you stop chest compressions?

After approximately 30 seconds of well-coordinated chest compressions and ventilation, you should stop compressions long enough to determine the heart rate again. If you can feel the pulse easily at the base of the cord, you will not need to stop ventilation; otherwise, you will need to stop both compressions and ventilation for a few seconds to allow you to listen to the chest with a stethoscope.

If the heart rate is now above 60 bpm, then

You can discontinue chest compressions, but continue positive-pressure ventilation now at the more rapid rate of 40 to 60 breaths per minute. You should not continue chest compressions, since the cardiac output is probably adequate and the compressions may decrease the effectiveness of the positive-pressure ventilation.

Once the heart rate rises above 100 bpm and the baby begins to breathe spontaneously, you should withdraw positive-pressure ventilation slowly, as described in Lesson 3, and move the baby to the nursery for post-resuscitation care.

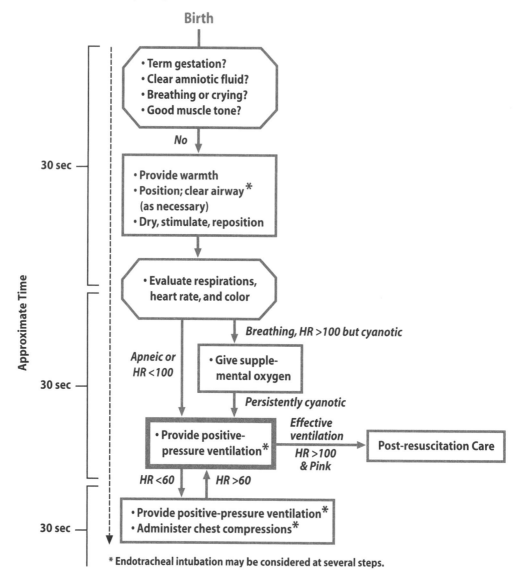

What do you do if the baby is *not* improving?

While chest compressions and positive-pressure ventilation are being delivered, there is a higher likelihood that air will enter the stomach, compared with ventilation alone. Therefore, unless you have already done so, it now may be advisable to pass an orogastric tube to vent the stomach. Also, many individuals will have chosen to insert an endotracheal tube by this time to eliminate the risk of stomach inflation and to improve the efficacy of ventilation.

While you are administering chest compressions and coordinated ventilation, continue to ask yourself the following questions:

- Is chest movement adequate? (Have you considered or performed endotracheal intubation? If so, is the endotracheal tube in the correct position?)
- Is supplemental oxygen being given?
- Is the depth of chest compression approximately one third of the diameter of the chest?
- Are the chest compressions and ventilation well coordinated?

If the heart rate remains below 60 bpm, then you should insert an umbilical catheter and give epinephrine, as described in Lesson 6.

As illustrated in Case 4 at the beginning of this lesson, by this point in a resuscitation you most likely will have intubated the trachea. The technique of endotracheal intubation will be described in Lesson 5.

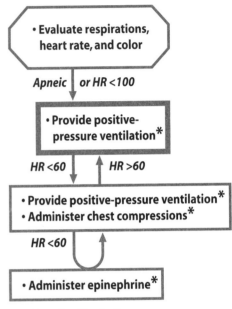

Key Points

1. Chest compressions are indicated when the heart rate remains less than 60 beats per minute, despite 30 seconds of effective positive-pressure ventilation.

2. Chest compressions

   - Compress the heart against the spine.

   - Increase intrathoracic pressure.

   - Circulate blood to the vital organs, including the brain.

3. There are 2 acceptable techniques for chest compressions—the thumb technique and the 2-finger technique—but the thumb technique usually is preferred.

4. Locate the correct area for compressions by running your fingers along the lower edge of the rib cage until you locate the xyphoid. Then place your thumbs or fingers on the sternum, above the xyphoid and on a line connecting the nipples.

5. To ensure proper rate of chest compressions and ventilation, the compressor repeats "One-and-Two-and-Three-and-Breathe-and…."

6. During chest compressions, the breathing rate is 30 breaths per minute and the compression rate is 90 compressions per minute. This equals 120 "events" per minute. One cycle of 3 compressions and 1 breath takes 2 seconds.

7. During chest compressions, ensure that

   - Chest movement is adequate during ventilation.

   - Supplemental oxygen is being used.

   - Compression depth is one third the diameter of the chest.

   - Pressure is released fully to permit chest recoil during relaxation phase of chest compression

   - Thumbs or fingers remain in contact with the chest at all times.

   - Duration of the downward stroke of the compression is shorter than duration of the release.

   - Chest compressions and ventilation are well coordinated.

8. After 30 seconds of chest compressions and ventilation, check the heart rate. If the heart rate is

   - Greater than 60 beats per minute, discontinue compressions and continue ventilation at 40 to 60 breaths per minute.

   - Greater than 100 beats per minute, discontinue compressions and gradually discontinue ventilation if the newborn is breathing spontaneously.

   - Less than 60 beats per minute, intubate the newborn, if not already done, and give epinephrine, preferably intravenously. Intubation provides a more reliable method of continuing ventilation.

Lesson 4 Review

(The answers follow.)

1. A newborn is apneic and blue. Her airway is cleared, and she is stimulated. At 30 seconds, positive-pressure ventilation is begun. At 60 seconds, her heart rate is 80 beats per minute. Chest compressions (should) (should not) be started. Positive-pressure ventilation (should) (should not) continue.

2. A newborn is apneic and blue. She remains apneic, despite having her airway cleared, being stimulated, and receiving 30 seconds of positive-pressure ventilation. At 60 seconds, her heart rate is 40 beats per minute. Chest compressions (should) (should not) be started. Positive-pressure ventilation (should) (should not) continue.

3. During the compression phase of chest compressions, the sternum compresses the heart, which causes blood to be pumped from the heart into the (veins) (arteries). In the release phase, blood enters the heart from the (veins) (arteries).

4. Mark the area on this baby (at right) where you would apply chest compressions.

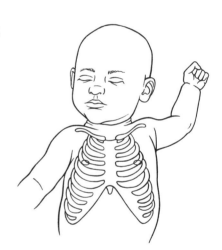

5. The preferred method of delivering chest compressions is the (thumb) (2-finger) technique.

6. If you anticipate that the baby will need medication by the umbilical route, it may be easier to deliver chest compressions with the (thumb) (2-finger) technique.

7. The correct depth of chest compressions is approximately

    A. One fourth of the anterior-posterior diameter of the chest

    B. One third of the anterior-posterior diameter of the chest

    C. One half of the anterior-posterior diameter of the chest

8. Which drawing shows the correct release motion?

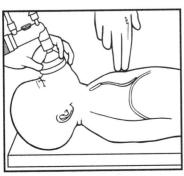

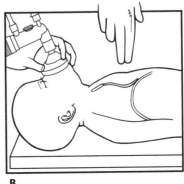

A.   **B.**

Lesson 4 Review — *continued*
(The answers follow.)

9. What phrase is used to time and coordinate chest compressions and ventilation? _____.

10. The ratio of chest compressions to ventilation is _____ to _____.

11. During positive-pressure ventilation without chest compressions, the rate of breaths per minute should be _____ to _____ breaths per minute.

12. During positive-pressure ventilation with chest compressions, the rate of "events" per minute should be _____ "events" per minute.

13. The count "One-and-Two-and-Three-and-Breathe-and" should take about _____ seconds.

14. A baby has required ventilation and chest compressions. After 30 seconds of chest compressions, you stop and count **8 heartbeats in 6 seconds.** The baby's heart rate is now _____ beats per minute. You should (continue) (stop) chest compressions.

15. A baby has required chest compressions and is being ventilated with bag and mask. The chest is not moving well. You stop and count **4 heartbeats in 6 seconds.** The baby's heart rate is now _____ beats per minute. You may want to consider _____, _____, and _____.

16. Complete the chart.

A. _____

_____

_____

B. _____

_____

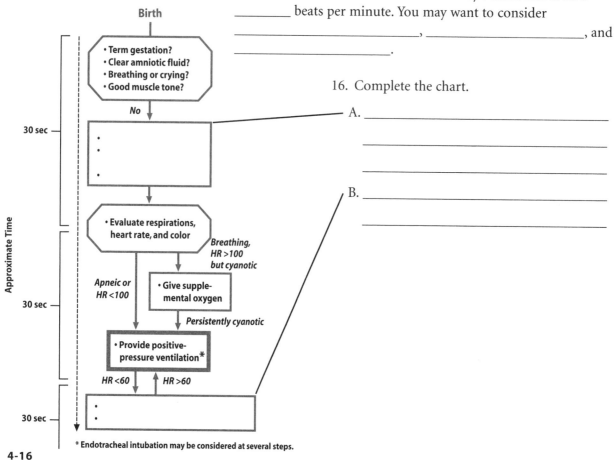

Birth

• Term gestation?
• Clear amniotic fluid?
• Breathing or crying?
• Good muscle tone?

No

30 sec

• :
• :
• :

• Evaluate respirations, heart rate, and color

Breathing, HR >100 but cyanotic

Apneic or HR <100

• Give supple-mental oxygen

30 sec

Persistently cyanotic

• Provide positive-pressure ventilation*

HR <60   HR >60

30 sec

• :
• :

Approximate Time

* Endotracheal intubation may be considered at several steps.

Answers to Questions

1. Chest compressions **should not** be started. Positive-pressure ventilation **should** continue.

2. Chest compressions **should** be started. Positive-pressure ventilation **should** continue.

3. Blood is pumped into the **arteries** during the compression phase and from the **veins** during the release phase.

4. Compression area

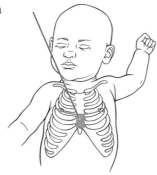

5. The preferred method of delivering chest compressions is the **thumb** technique.

6. The **2-finger** technique may be easier if medications will be given by the umbilical route.

7. The correct depth of chest compressions is approximately **one third of the anterior-posterior diameter of the chest** (B).

8. Drawing **A** is correct (fingers remain in contact during release).

9. "One-and-Two-and-Three-and-Breathe-and …"

10. The ratio is **3:1.**

11. The rate of ventilation without chest compressions should be **40 to 60** breaths per minute.

12. There should be **120** "events" per minute during chest compressions.

13. The count "One-and-Two-and-Three-and-Breathe-and" should take about **2** seconds.

14. Eight heartbeats in 6 seconds is **80** beats per minute. You should **stop** chest compressions.

15. Four heartbeats in 6 seconds is **40** beats per minute. You may want to consider **endotracheal intubation, insertion of an umbilical catheter,** and **administration of epinephrine.**

16. A.
   - **Provide warmth**
   - **Position; clear airway***
     (as necessary)
   - **Dry, stimulate, reposition**

   B.
   - **Provide positive-pressure ventilation***
   - **Administer chest compressions***

Performance Checklist

Lesson 4 — Chest Compressions

Instructor: The learner should be instructed to talk through the procedure as it is demonstrated. Judge the performance of each step and check (✓) the box when the action is completed correctly. If done incorrectly, circle the box so that you can discuss that step later. At several points, you will need to provide information concerning the condition of the baby.

Learner: To successfully complete this checklist, you should be able to perform all the steps and make all the correct decisions in the procedure. You should talk through the procedure as you perform it.

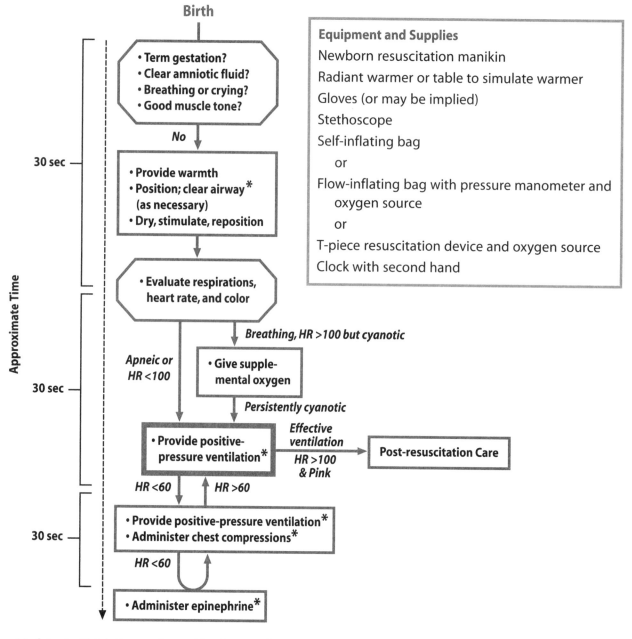

* Endotracheal intubation may be considered at several steps.

Performance Checklist

Lesson 4 — Chest Compressions

Name _____ Instructor _____ Date _____

This performance checklist includes responsibilities for 2 learners: one who ventilates the baby and one who provides chest compressions. If only one learner is being evaluated, the instructor should assume the role of the other learner. The location of the check box indicates which learner is responsible for each activity. Each learner should demonstrate skills in both roles, and each learner must serve as Learner #1 twice to demonstrate both methods of performing chest compressions.

Instructor's questions are in quotes. Learner's questions and correct responses are in bold type. Instructor should check boxes as the learner answers correctly.

"This baby born at term has been provided warmth, positioned, suctioned, dried, and given tactile stimulation. He remains apneic."

Learner #1   ## Learner #2

Initiates bag-and-mask ventilation with 100% oxygen   ☐

After 30 seconds, asks for heart rate check   ☐

☐ **Checks the heart rate by palpation for exactly 6 seconds**

"You detect 4 beats in 6 seconds."

☐ **Announces heart rate of 40 bpm and indicates need for chest compressions**

☐ **Locates appropriate position on lower one third of sternum**

☐ **Provides firm support for baby's back**

	2-finger technique	Thumb technique
	☐ **Uses fingertips of middle and index or ring fingers**	☐ **Uses distal portion of both thumbs**

☐ **Compresses sternum approximately one third of the anterior-posterior diameter of chest**

☐ **Keeps fingertips/thumbs on sternum during release**

☐ **Brings tempo to approximately 2 compressions per second with a pause after every third compression for ventilation; counts cadence** ("One-and-Two-and-Three-and-Breathe-and...")

Learner #1   Learner #2

☐   Ventilates during the pause after every third compression

☐   Provides adequate ventilation pressure and head/mask placement to achieve adequate chest movement

☐   Checks the heart rate by palpation for exactly 6 seconds after 30 seconds of chest compressions

"You detect no pulsations."

☐   Learner #2 ceases ventilation while Learner #1 checks the heart rate by auscultation   ☐

"You detect 5 beats in 6 seconds."

☐   Announces heart rate of 50 bpm and resumes chest compressions

☐   Resumes ventilation immediately after heart rate check and considers

- Is chest movement adequate?

- Is supplemental oxygen being given?

- Is the depth of chest compression approximately one third the diameter of the chest?

- Are chest compressions and ventilation being well coordinated?

- Are endotracheal intubation and/or epinephrine indicated?

☐   Checks heart rate by palpation for exactly 6 seconds 30 seconds after previous heart rate check

"You detect 9 beats in 6 seconds."

☐   Announces heart rate of 90 bpm and discontinues chest compressions

☐   Continues ventilation   ☐

Overall performance, judged after performing both roles

☐ Correctly coordinated chest compressions with ventilation

☐ Correctly stated whether chest compressions should be stopped or continued, depending on heart rate

☐ Correctly performed thumb technique

☐ Correctly performed 2-finger technique

☐ Correctly evaluated heart rate at appropriate times (first palpated cord then, if necessary, ceased ventilation and listened to chest with stethoscope)

☐ Speed—carried out action without undue delay

Endotracheal Intubation

In Lesson 5 you will learn

- The indications for endotracheal intubation during resuscitation

- How to select and prepare the appropriate equipment for endotracheal intubation

- How to use the laryngoscope to insert an endotracheal tube

- How to determine if the endotracheal tube is in the trachea

- How to use the endotracheal tube to suction meconium from the trachea

- How to use the endotracheal tube to administer positive-pressure ventilation

When is endotracheal intubation required?

Endotracheal intubation may be performed at various points during a resuscitation as indicated by the asterisks in the flow diagram. Case 2 (Lesson 2, page 2-3) illustrated one such point, where the trachea was intubated to suction meconium. Case 4 (Lesson 4, page 4-2) illustrated another point, where bag-and-mask ventilation was ineffective and the trachea was intubated to improve ventilation and to facilitate coordination of ventilation and chest compressions. The timing of intubation is determined by many factors, one of which is the intubation skill of the resuscitator. People who are not adept at intubation should call for help and focus on providing effective ventilation with a positive-pressure device and mask, rather than spending valuable time trying to intubate. Other factors influencing the timing of intubation include the following:

- If there is meconium and the baby has depressed respirations, muscle tone, or heart rate, you need to intubate the trachea as the very first step, before any other resuscitation measures are started.

- If positive-pressure ventilation is not resulting in adequate clinical improvement, if there is not good chest movement, or if the need for positive-pressure ventilation lasts beyond a few minutes, you may decide to intubate to improve the efficacy and ease of assisted ventilation.

- If chest compressions are necessary, intubating may facilitate coordination of chest compressions and ventilation and maximize the efficiency of each positive-pressure breath.

- As you will learn in the next lesson, if epinephrine is required to stimulate the heart, one common route to administer the epinephrine is directly into the trachea while intravenous access is being established. This, too, will require endotracheal intubation.

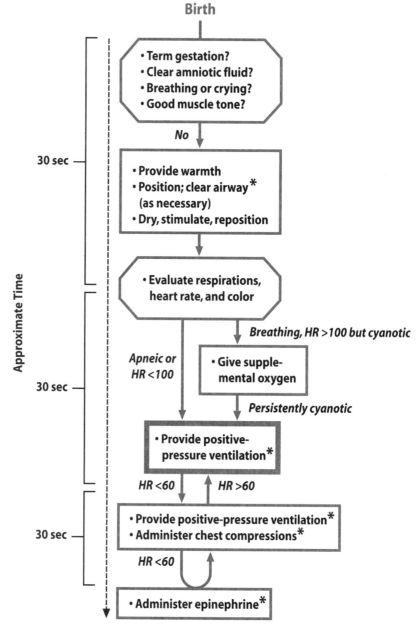

* Endotracheal intubation may be considered at several steps.

There are also some special indications for endotracheal intubation, such as for extreme prematurity, surfactant administration, and suspected diaphragmatic hernia. These indications are discussed in Lessons 7 and 8.

What alternatives are there to endotracheal intubation?

Masks that fit over the laryngeal inlet (Figure 5.1) have been shown to be an effective alternative for assisting ventilation when positive-pressure ventilation by bag and mask or mask and T-piece resuscitator is ineffective and attempts at intubation are not feasible or are unsuccessful. However, there are limited data about the use of laryngeal mask airways for neonatal resuscitation. Experience with laryngeal masks in preterm newborns and in meconium-stained newborns is even more limited. If your hospital uses laryngeal mask airways for neonatal resuscitation, you will need to stock them on your resuscitation trays and personnel will require special training in their use. The details of laryngeal mask insertion are covered in the Appendix to this lesson.

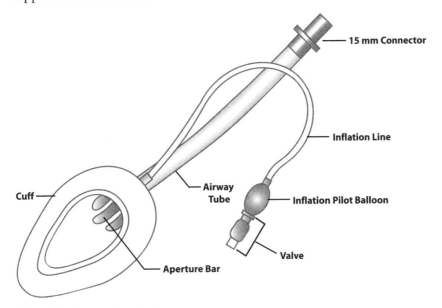

Figure 5.1. Laryngeal mask airway

What equipment and supplies are needed?

The supplies and equipment necessary to perform endotracheal intubation should be kept together and readily available. Each delivery room, nursery, and emergency department should have at least one complete set of the following items (Figure 5.2):

1. Laryngoscope with an extra set of batteries and extra bulbs.

2. Blades: No. 1 (term newborn), No. 0 (preterm newborn), No. 00 (optional for extremely preterm newborn). Straight rather than curved blades are preferred.

3. Endotracheal tubes with inside diameters of 2.5, 3.0, 3.5, and 4.0 mm.

4. Stylet (optional) that fits into the endotracheal tubes in this kit.

5. Carbon dioxide (CO_2) monitor or detector.

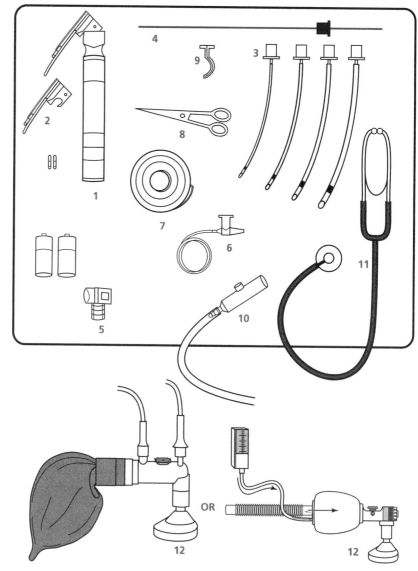

Figure 5.2. Neonatal resuscitation equipment and supplies

6. Suction setup with 10F or larger suction catheter, plus sizes 5F or 6F and 8F for suctioning the endotracheal tube.

7. Roll of tape, 1/2 or 3/4 inch, or endotracheal tube securing device.

8. Scissors.

9. Oral airway.

10. Meconium aspirator.

11. Stethoscope (neonatal head preferred).

12. Positive-pressure device, pressure gauge (optional for self-inflating bags), and oxygen tubing. Self-inflating bag must have oxygen reservoir.

This equipment should be stored together in a clearly marked container and placed in a readily accessible location.

Intubation is best performed as a clean procedure. The endotracheal tubes and stylet should be clean and protected from contamination. The laryngoscope blades and handle should be cleaned after each use.

What kind of endotracheal tubes are best to use?

Endotracheal tubes are supplied in sterile packages and should be handled with clean technique. They should be of uniform diameter throughout the length of the tube, not tapered near the tip (Figure 5.3). One disadvantage of the tapered tube is that, during intubation, your view of the tracheal opening is easily obstructed by the wide part of the tube. Also, tubes with shoulders are more likely to become obstructed and cause trauma to the vocal cords.

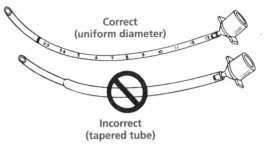

Figure 5.3. Endotracheal tubes with uniform diameter are preferred for newborns

Most endotracheal tubes for newborns have a black line near the tip of the tube, which is called a "vocal cord guide" (Figure 5.4). Such tubes are meant to be inserted so that the vocal cord guide is placed at the level of the vocal cords. This usually positions the tip of the tube above the bifurcation of the trachea (carina).

The length of the trachea in a premature newborn is less than that of a term newborn—3 cm versus 5 to 6 cm. Therefore, the smaller the tube, the closer the vocal cord guide is to the tip of the tube. However, there is some variability among tube manufacturers regarding the placement of the vocal cord guide.

Although tubes are available with cuffs at the level of the vocal cord guide, cuffs are not recommended when endotracheal intubation is required for resuscitation of newborns.

Most endotracheal tubes made for newborns come with centimeter markings along the tube, identifying the distance from the tip of the tube. Later, you will learn to use these markings to identify the appropriate depth of insertion of the tube.

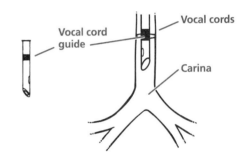

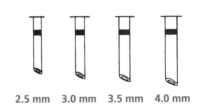

2.5 mm   3.0 mm   3.5 mm   4.0 mm

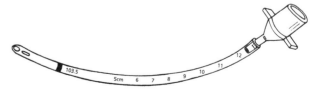

Figure 5.4. Characteristics of endotracheal tubes used for neonatal resuscitation

How do you prepare the endotracheal tube for use?

Select the appropriate-sized tube.

Tube Size (mm) (inside diameter)	Weight (g)	Gestational Age (wks)
2.5	Below 1,000	Below 28
3.0	1,000–2,000	28–34
3.5	2,000–3,000	34–38
3.5–4.0	Above 3,000	Above 38

Table 5-1. Endotracheal tube size for babies of various weights and gestational ages

Time is limited once resuscitation is underway. Therefore, preparation of equipment before an anticipated high-risk delivery is important.

The approximate size of the endotracheal tube is determined from the baby's weight. Table 5-1 gives the tube size for various weight and gestational age categories. Study the table. Later you will be asked to recall the suggested tube size for babies of various weights. It may be helpful to post the table in each delivery room, on or near the radiant warmers.

Consider cutting the tube to a shorter length.
Many endotracheal tubes come from the manufacturer much longer than necessary for orotracheal use. The extra length will increase resistance to airflow.

Some clinicians find it helpful to shorten the endotracheal tube before insertion (Figure 5.5). The endotracheal tube may be shortened to 13 to 15* cm to make it easier to handle during intubation and to lessen the chance of inserting the tube too far. A 13- to 15-cm tube will provide enough tube extending beyond the baby's lips for you to adjust the depth of insertion, if necessary, and to properly secure the tube to the face. Remove the connector (note that the connection to the tube may be tight), and then cut the tube diagonally to make it easier to reinsert the connector.

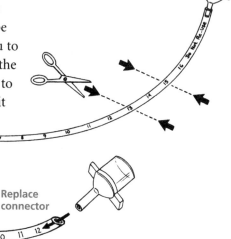

Replace the endotracheal tube connector. The fitting should be tight so that the connector does not inadvertently separate during insertion or use. Ensure that the connector and tube are properly aligned so that kinking of the tube is avoided. Connectors are made to fit a specific-sized tube. They cannot be interchanged among tubes of different sizes.

Replace connector

Figure 5.5. Process of cutting endotracheal tube to length before insertion

Others prefer to leave the tube long initially and then cut the tube to length after insertion if it is decided to leave it in place for longer than the immediate resuscitation.

*Note: The 15-cm length may be preferred to accommodate some types of endotracheal tube securing devices.

Consider using a stylet (optional).

Some people find it helpful to place a stylet through the endotracheal tube to provide rigidity and curvature to the tube, thus facilitating intubation (Figure 5.6). When inserting the stylet, it is essential that

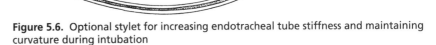

- The tip does not protrude from the end or side hole of the endotracheal tube (to avoid trauma to the tissues).

- The stylet is secured so that it cannot advance farther into the tube during intubation.

Figure 5.6. Optional stylet for increasing endotracheal tube stiffness and maintaining curvature during intubation

Although many find the stylet helpful, others find the stiffness of the tube alone adequate. Use of a stylet is optional and depends on the operator's preference and skill.

 Caution: When stylets are reused, the plastic coating may have torn and they may have bends in them that make them fit very tightly in the endotracheal tube. Before using, check to make certain that the stylet is intact and can be removed from the tube easily.

How do you prepare the laryngoscope and additional supplies?

Select blade and attach to handle.

First, select the appropriate-sized blade and attach it to the laryngoscope handle.

- No. 0 for preterm newborns

- No. 1 for term newborns

Check light.

Next, turn on the light by clicking the blade into the "open" position to determine that the batteries and bulb are working. Check to see that the bulb is screwed in tightly to ensure that it will not flicker or fall out during the procedure.

Prepare suction equipment.

Suction equipment should be available and ready for use.

- Adjust the suction source to 100 mm Hg by increasing or decreasing the level of suction while occluding the end of the suction tubing.

- Connect a 10F (or larger) suction catheter to the suction tubing so that it is available to suction secretions from the mouth and nose.

- Smaller suction catheters (5F, 6F, or 8F, depending on the size of the endotracheal tube) should be available for suctioning the tube if it becomes necessary to leave the endotracheal tube in place. Appropriate sizes are listed in Table 5-2.

Endotracheal Tube Size	Catheter Size
2.5	5F or 6F
3.0	6F or 8F
3.5	8F
4.0	8F or 10F

Table 5-2. Suction catheter size for endotracheal tubes of various inner diameters

Prepare device for administering positive pressure.

A resuscitation bag and mask or T-piece resuscitator capable of providing 90% to 100% oxygen should be on hand to ventilate the baby between intubation attempts or if intubation is unsuccessful. The resuscitation device without the mask will be required to ventilate the baby after intubation, initially to check tube placement and subsequently to provide continued ventilation, if necessary. Check the operation of the device as described in Lesson 3.

Turn on oxygen.

The oxygen tubing should be connected to an oxygen source and be available to deliver up to 100% free-flow oxygen and to connect to the resuscitation device. The oxygen flow should be set at 5 to 10 L/min.

Get stethoscope.

A stethoscope will be needed to check for breath sounds.

Cut tape or prepare stabilizer.

Cut a strip of adhesive tape to secure the tube to the face, or prepare an endotracheal tube holder, if used at your hospital.

Review

(The answers are in the preceding section and at the end of the lesson.)

1. A newborn with meconium and depressed respirations (will) (will not) require suctioning by endotracheal intubation before positive-pressure ventilation is administered.

2. A newborn receiving ventilation by bag and mask is not improving after 2 minutes of apparently good technique. The heart rate is not rising and there is poor chest movement. Endotracheal intubation (should) (should not) be considered.

3. For babies weighing less than 1,000 g, the inside diameter of the endotracheal tube should be _____ mm.

4. The blade of a laryngoscope for preterm newborns should be No. _____. The blade for term newborns should be No. _____.

What anatomy do you need to know to insert the tube properly?

The anatomic landmarks that relate to intubation are labeled in Figures 5.7 through 5.9. Study the relative position of these landmarks, using all the figures, because each is important to your understanding of the procedure.

1. **Epiglottis**—A lidlike structure overhanging the entrance to the trachea

2. **Vallecula**—A pouch formed by the base of the tongue and the epiglottis

3. **Esophagus**—The food passageway extending from the throat to the stomach

4. **Cricoid**—Lower portion of the cartilage of the larynx

5. **Glottis**—The opening of the larynx leading to the trachea, flanked by the vocal cords

6. **Vocal cords**—Mucous membrane-covered ligaments on both sides of the glottis

7. **Trachea**—The windpipe or air passageway, extending from the throat to the main bronchi

8. **Main bronchi**—The 2 air passageways leading from the trachea to the lungs

9. **Carina**—Where the trachea branches into the 2 main bronchi

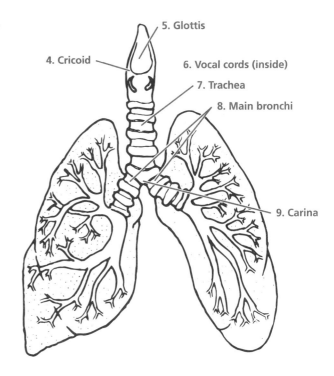

Figure 5.7. Anatomy of the airway

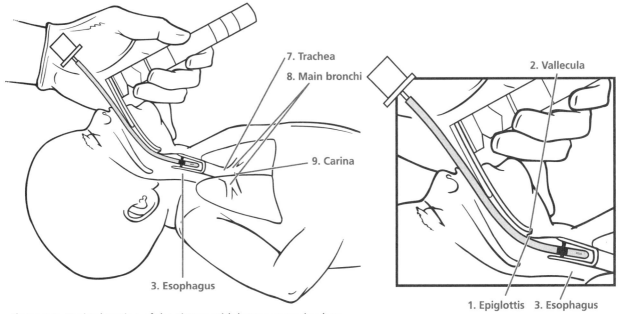

Figure 5.8. Sagittal section of the airway, with laryngoscope in place

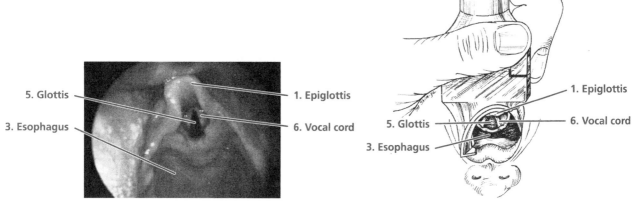

5. Glottis — ... — 1. Epiglottis

3. Esophagus — ... — 6. Vocal cord

1. Epiglottis

5. Glottis — ... — 6. Vocal cord

3. Esophagus

Figure 5.9. Photograph and drawing of laryngoscopic view of glottis and surrounding structures

From Klaus M. Fanaroff A.
Care of the High Risk Neonate.
Philadelphia, PA: WB Saunders, 1996

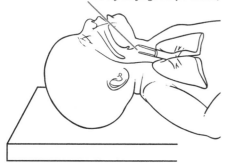

Correct — Line of sight clear (tongue will be lifted by laryngoscope blade)

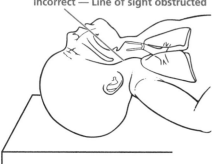

Incorrect — Line of sight obstructed

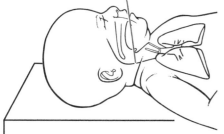

Incorrect — Line of sight obstructed

Figure 5.10. Correct (top) and incorrect (middle and bottom) positioning for intubation

How should you position the newborn to make intubation easiest?

The correct position of the newborn for intubation is the same as for bag-and-mask ventilation—on a flat surface with the head in a midline position and the neck slightly extended. It may be helpful to place a roll under the baby's shoulders to maintain slight extension of the neck.

This "sniffing" position aligns the trachea for optimal viewing by allowing a straight line of sight into the glottis once the laryngoscope has been properly placed (Figure 5.10).

It is important not to hyperextend the neck, because this will raise the glottis above your line of sight and narrow the trachea.

If there is too much flexion of the head toward the chest, you will be viewing the posterior pharynx and may not be able to directly visualize the glottis.

How do you hold the laryngoscope?

Turn on the laryngoscope light and hold the laryngoscope in your *left* hand, between your thumb and first 2 or 3 fingers, with the blade pointing away from you (Figure 5.11). One or 2 fingers should be left free to rest on the baby's face to provide stability.

The laryngoscope is designed to be held in the *left* hand—by both right- and left-handed persons. If held in the right hand, the closed curved part of the blade will block your view of the glottis, as well as make insertion of the endotracheal tube impossible.

How do you visualize the glottis and insert the tube?

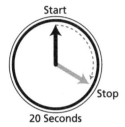

Start

Stop

20 Seconds

The next few steps will be described in detail. However, during an actual resuscitation, they need to be completed very quickly—within approximately 20 seconds.* The baby will not be ventilated during this process, so quick action is essential. Color photos of this procedure can be found on page C in the center section of the book.

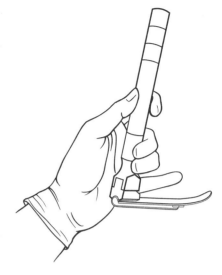

Figure 5.11. Correct hand position when holding a laryngoscope for neonatal intubation

First, stabilize the baby's head with your right hand (Figure 5.12). It may be helpful to have a second person hold the head in the desired "sniffing" position. Free-flow oxygen should be delivered throughout the procedure.

*Note: Although this program recommends a goal of 20 seconds to perform endotracheal intubation, studies have shown that a somewhat longer time may be required in clinical practice. The important concept is that the procedure be accomplished as quickly as possible. If the patient appears to be compromised, it is usually preferable to stop, resume positive-pressure ventilation with a mask, and then try again.

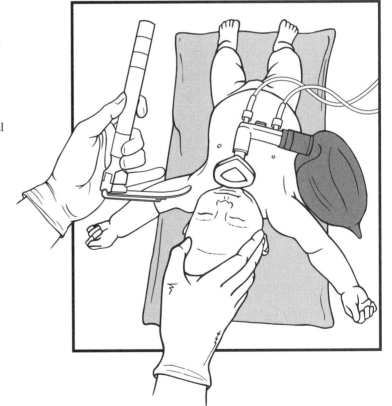

Figure 5.12. Preparing to insert the larynogoscope

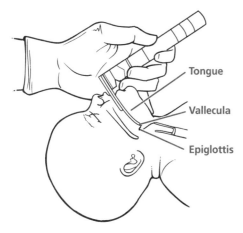

Figure 5.13. Landmarks for placement of the laryngoscope

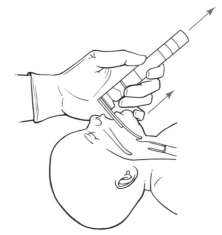

Figure 5.14. Lifting the laryngoscope blade to expose the opening of the larynx

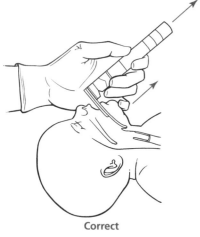

Correct

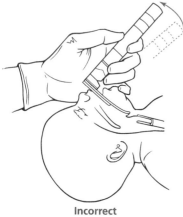

Incorrect

Figure 5.15. Correct (top) and incorrect (bottom) method for lifting the laryngoscope blade to expose the larynx

Second, slide the laryngoscope blade over the right side of the tongue, pushing the tongue to the left side of the mouth, and advance the blade until the tip lies in the vallecula, just beyond the base of the tongue (Figure 5.13). You may need to use your right index finger to open the baby's mouth to make it easier to insert the laryngoscope.

Note: Although this lesson describes placing the tip of the blade in the vallecula, some prefer to place it directly on the epiglottis, *gently* compressing the epiglottis against the base of the tongue.

Third, lift the blade slightly, thus lifting the tongue out of the way to expose the pharyngeal area (Figure 5.14).

When lifting the blade, raise the *entire* blade by pulling up in the direction the handle is pointing (Figure 5.15).

Do not elevate the tip of the blade by using a rocking motion and pulling the handle toward you.

Rocking rather than elevating the tip of the blade will not produce the view of the glottis you desire and will put excessive pressure on the alveolar ridge.

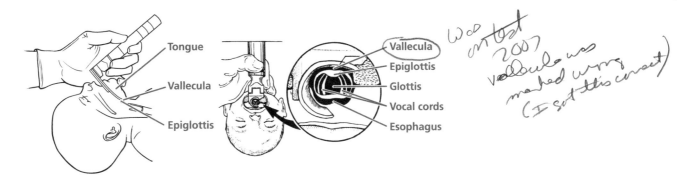

Figure 5.16. Identification of landmarks before placing endotracheal tube through glottis

Fourth, look for landmarks (Figure 5.16). (Also, see color Figures C-2a, C-2b, C-2c, and C2d in the center of the book.)

If the tip of the blade is correctly positioned in the vallecula, you should see the epiglottis at the top, with the glottic opening below. You also should see the vocal cords appearing as vertical stripes on each side of the glottis or as an inverted letter "V" (Figure 5.9).

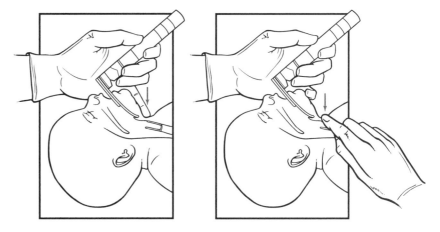

Figure 5.17. Improving visualization with pressure applied to larynx by intubator (left) or by an assistant (right)

If these structures are not immediately visible, quickly adjust the blade until the structures come into view. Applying downward pressure to the cricoid (the cartilage that covers the larynx) may help bring the glottis into view (Figure 5.17). The pressure may be applied with your own little finger or by an assistant.

Suctioning of secretions may help to improve your view (Figure 5.18). Inadequate visualization of the glottis is the most common reason for unsuccessful intubation.

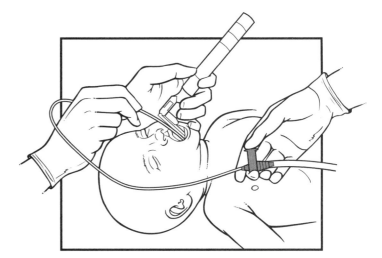

Figure 5.18. Suctioning of secretions

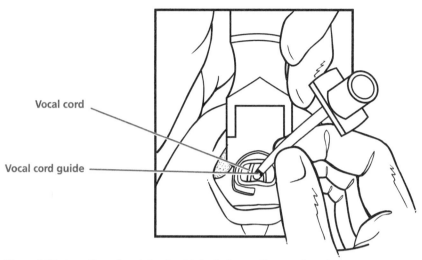

Figure 5.19. Insertion of endotracheal tube between the vocal cords

Fifth, insert the tube (Figure 5.19).

Holding the tube in your right hand, introduce it into the right side of the baby's mouth, with the curve of the tube lying in the horizontal plane. This will prevent the tube from blocking your view of the glottis.

Keep the glottis in view and, when the vocal cords are apart, insert the tip of the endotracheal tube until the vocal cord guide is at the level of the cords.

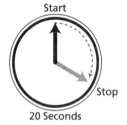

If the cords are together, wait for them to open. Do not touch the closed cords with the tip of the tube because it may cause spasm of the cords. Never try to force the tube between closed cords. If the cords do not open within 20 seconds, stop and ventilate with a bag and mask. After the heart rate and color have improved, you can try again.

Be careful to insert the tube only so far as to place the vocal cord guide at the level of the vocal cords (Figure 5.20). This positions the tube in the trachea approximately halfway between the vocal cords and the carina.

Note the markings on the tube that align with the baby's lip.

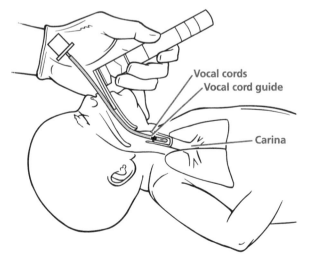

Figure 5.20. Correct depth of insertion of endotracheal tube

Sixth, stabilize the tube with one hand, and remove the laryngoscope with the other (Figure 5.21).

With the right hand held against the face, hold the tube *firmly* at the lips and/or use a finger to hold the tube against the baby's hard palate. Use your left hand to *carefully* remove the laryngoscope without displacing the tube.

If a stylet was used, remove it from the endotracheal tube—again be careful to hold the tube in place while you do so (Figure 5.22).

> ! **Although it is important to hold the tube firmly, be careful not to press the tube so tightly that the tube becomes compressed and obstructs airflow.**

You are now ready to use the tube for the reason you inserted it.

- If the purpose is to **suction meconium,** then use the tube as described on the next page.
- If the purpose is to **ventilate the baby,** then quickly attach a ventilation bag or T-piece resuscitator to the tube, take steps to be certain the tube is in the trachea, and resume positive-pressure ventilation with 100% oxygen (Figure 5.23).

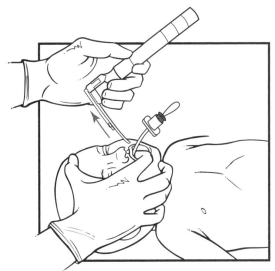

Figure 5.21. Stabilizing the tube while laryngoscope is withdrawn

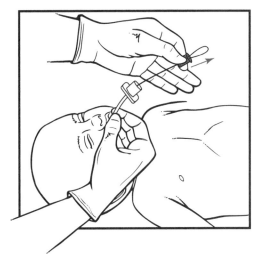

Figure 5.22. Removing stylet from endotracheal tube

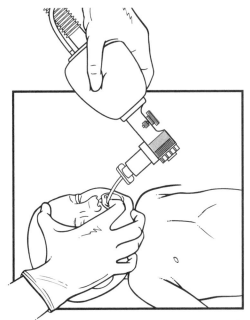

Figure 5.23. Resuming positive-pressure ventilation after endotracheal intubation

What do you do next if the tube was inserted to suction meconium?

As described in Lesson 2, if there is meconium in the amniotic fluid and the baby has depressed muscle tone, depressed respirations, or a heart rate less than 100 beats per minute (bpm) (ie, not vigorous), the trachea should be intubated and suctioned.

As soon as the endotracheal tube has been inserted and the stylet, if used, has been removed,

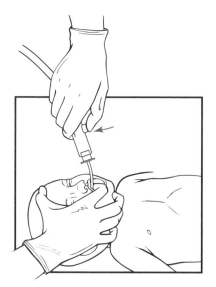

Figure 5.24. Suctioning meconium from trachea using an endotracheal tube, meconium aspiration device, and suction tubing connected to a suction source

- Connect the endotracheal tube to a meconium aspirator, which has been connected to a suction source (Figure 5.24). Several alternative types of meconium aspirators are commercially available, some of which include the endotracheal tube as part of the device.

- Occlude the suction-control port on the aspirator to apply suction to the endotracheal tube, and gradually withdraw the tube as you continue suctioning any meconium that may be in the trachea.

- Repeat intubation and suction as necessary until little or no additional meconium is recovered or until the baby's heart rate indicates that positive-pressure ventilation is needed.

For how long do you try to suction meconium?

Judgment is required when suctioning meconium. You have learned to suction the trachea only if the meconium-stained baby has depressed respirations or muscle tone, or has a heart rate less than 100 bpm. Therefore, at the time you begin to suction the trachea, it is likely that the baby will already be significantly compromised and will eventually need resuscitation. You will need to delay resuscitation for a few seconds while you suction meconium, but you do not want to delay longer than absolutely necessary.

The following are a few guidelines:

- Do not apply suction to the endotracheal tube for longer than 3 to 5 seconds as you withdraw the tube.

- If no meconium is recovered, don't repeat the procedure; proceed with resuscitation.

- If you recover meconium with the first suction, check the heart rate. If the baby does not have significant bradycardia, reintubate and suction again. If the heart rate is low, you may decide to administer positive pressure without repeating the procedure.

If you intubated to ventilate the baby, how do you check to be sure that the tube is in the trachea?

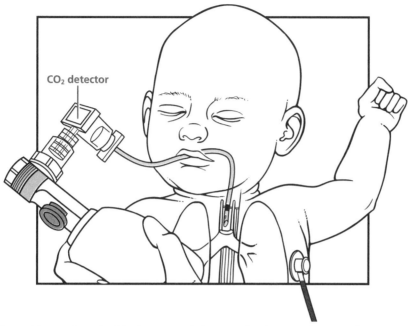

CO₂ detector

Figure 5.25. Carbon dioxide detector will change color during exhalation if endotracheal tube is in the trachea

Watching the tube pass between the cords, watching for chest movement following application of positive pressure, and listening for breath sounds are all helpful signs that the tube is in the trachea rather than the esophagus. However, these signs can be misleading. An increasing heart rate and CO_2 detection are the primary methods for confirming endotracheal tube placement (Figure 5.25).

There are 2 basic types of CO_2 detectors available.

- Colorimetric devices are connected to the endotracheal tube and change color in the presence of CO_2. (See color Figures D-1, D-2, and D-3 in the center of the book.)

- Capnographs rely on placement of a special electrode at the endotracheal tube connector. The capnograph then will display a specific CO_2 level and should read more than 2% to 3% CO_2 if the tube is in the trachea.

The colorimetric device is the most commonly used method.

As soon as you have inserted the endotracheal tube, connect a CO_2 detector and note the presence or absence of CO_2 during exhalation. If CO_2 is not detected after several positive-pressure breaths, consider removing the tube, resuming bag-and-mask ventilation, and repeating the intubation process as described on pages 5-10 through 5-15.

! **Caution: Babies with very poor cardiac output may exhale insufficient CO_2 to be detected reliably by CO_2 detectors.**

If the tube is positioned correctly, you also should observe the following:

- Improvement in heart rate and color
- Breath sounds audible over both lung fields but decreased or absent over the stomach (Figure 5.26)
- No gastric distention with ventilation
- Vapor condensing on the inside of the tube during exhalation
- Symmetrical movement of the chest with each breath

When listening to breath sounds, be sure to use a small stethoscope and place it laterally and high on the chest wall (in the axilla). A large stethoscope, or a stethoscope placed either too near the center or too low on the chest, may transmit sounds from the esophagus or stomach. Observe for absence of gastric distension and movement of both sides of the chest with each ventilated breath.

Listening for bilateral breath sounds and observing symmetrical chest movement with positive-pressure ventilation provide secondary confirmation of correct endotracheal tube placement in the airway with the tip of the tube positioned above the carina. A rapid increase in heart rate is indicative of effective positive-pressure ventilation.

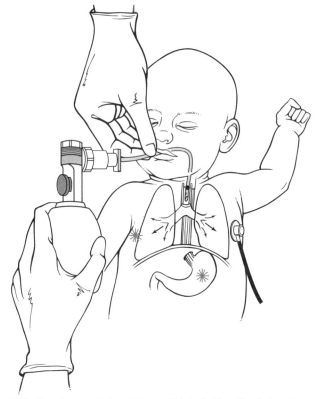

Figure 5.26. Breath sounds should be audible in both axillae but not over stomach (see asterisks)

 Be cautious when interpreting breath sounds in newborns. Because sounds are easily transmitted, those heard over the anterior portions of the chest may be coming from the stomach or esophagus. Breath sounds also can be transmitted to the abdomen.

What do you do if you suspect that the tube may *not* be in the trachea?

 Be certain that the tube is in the trachea. A misplaced tube is worse than having no tube at all.

The tube is likely not in the trachea if

- The newborn remains cyanotic and bradycardic despite positive-pressure ventilation.
- The CO_2 detector does not indicate presence of CO_2.
- You do not hear good breath sounds over the lungs.
- The abdomen appears to become distended.
- You do hear air noises over the stomach.
- There is no mist in the tube.
- The chest is not moving symmetrically with each positive-pressure breath.

If you suspect the tube is not in the trachea, you should do the following:

- Use your right hand to hold the tube in place while you use your left hand to reinsert the laryngoscope so that you can visualize the glottis and see if the tube is passing between the vocal cords.

and/or

- Remove the tube, use a resuscitation device and mask to stabilize the heart rate and color, and then repeat the intubation procedure.

Note: The CO_2 monitor may not change color if the cardiac output is very low or absent (eg, cardiac arrest). If there is no detectable heartbeat, do not use the CO_2 monitor as an indicator of correct or incorrect placement of the endotracheal tube.

u know if the tip of the tube is in the tion within the trachea?

correctly placed, the tip will be located in the midtrachea, ween the vocal cords and the carina. On the x-ray the tip sible at the level of the clavicles, or slightly below). If it is in too far, it generally will be down the right main and you will be ventilating only the right lung (Figure 5.28).

e is correctly placed and the lungs are inflating, you will hear unds of equal intensity on each side.

be is in too far, you will hear breath sounds that are louder on e than the other (usually the right). If that is the case, pull back e very slowly while listening to the left side of the chest. When be is pulled back and the tip reaches the carina, you should hear equal breath sounds.

You also can use the tip-to-lip measurement to estimate if the tube has been inserted the correct distance (Table 5-3). Adding 6 to the baby's weight in kilograms will give you a rough estimate of the correct distance from the tube tip to the vermilion border of the upper lip. (Note: This rule is unreliable in those babies who have congenital anomalies of the neck and mandible [eg, Robin syndrome].)

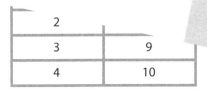

2	
3	9
4	10

Table 5-3. Estimated distance from tip of tube to baby's lip, based on baby's weight

*Babies weighing less than 750 g may require only 6 cm insertion.

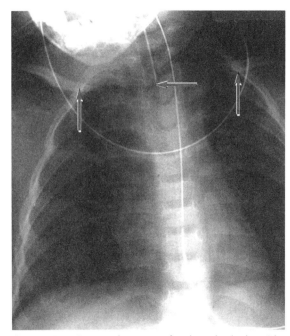

Figure 5.27. *Correct* placement of endotracheal tube with tip in midtrachea. The horizontal arrow points to the tip of the tube. The vertical arrows point to the clavicles

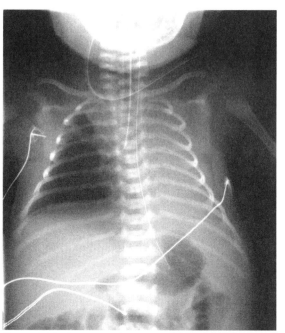

Figure 5.28. *Incorrect* placement of endotracheal tube with tip in right main bronchus. Note collapse of left lung

After you have ensured that the tube is in the correct position, take note of the centimeter marking that appears at the upper lip. This can help you maintain the appropriate depth of insertion (Figure 5.29).

If the tube is going to be left in place beyond the initial resuscitation, you should obtain a chest x-ray as a final confirmation that the tube is in the proper position.

For long-term positive-pressure ventilation, the tube also needs to be secured to the face. Description of this technique is beyond the scope of this program. If you did not previously shorten the tube, it would be appropriate to do so now. However, be prepared to reinsert the connector quickly, as you will be unable to attach the resuscitation bag or T-piece resuscitator until you do so.

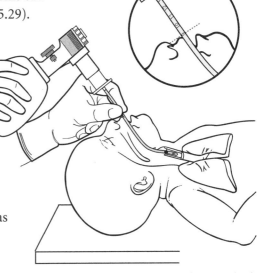

Figure 5.29. Measurement of endotracheal tube marking at the lip

How do you continue resuscitation while you intubate?

Unfortunately, you cannot continue most resuscitation actions while intubating.

- Ventilation must be discontinued because the bag and mask must be removed from the airway during the procedure.
- Chest compressions must be interrupted because the compressions cause movement and prevent you from seeing landmarks.

Therefore, make every effort to minimize the amount of hypoxia imposed during intubation. The following will be helpful:

- *Pre-oxygenate before attempting intubation.*
  Oxygenate the baby appropriately with resuscitation device and mask before beginning intubation and between repeated intubation attempts. This will not be possible when intubation is being performed for suctioning meconium or when a baby is being intubated to improve ineffective positive-pressure ventilation.

- *Deliver free-flow oxygen during intubation.*
  Hold 100% free-flow oxygen by the baby's face while the intubator is clearing the airway and visualizing the landmarks. Then, if the baby makes any spontaneous respiratory efforts during the procedure, he will breathe oxygen-enriched air.

- *Limit attempts to 20 seconds.*
  Don't try to intubate for longer than approximately 20 seconds. If you are unable to visualize the glottis and insert the tube within 20 seconds, remove the laryngoscope and attempt to oxygenate the baby with bag-and-mask ventilation using 100% oxygen. Ensure that the baby is stable, then try again.

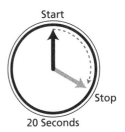

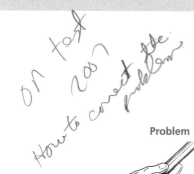

What can go wrong while you are trying to intubate?

You may have trouble visualizing the glottis (Figure 5.30).

Problem	Landmarks	Corrective Action

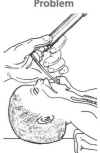 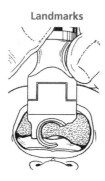 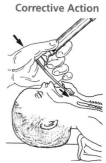

Laryngoscope not inserted far enough.	You see the tongue surrounding the blade.	Advance the blade farther.

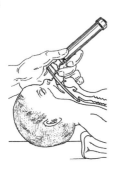 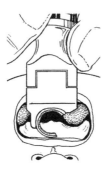 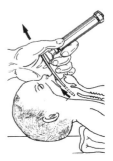

Laryngoscope inserted too far.	You see the walls of the esophagus surrounding the blade.	Withdraw the blade slowly until the epiglottis and glottis are seen.

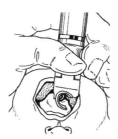 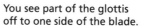 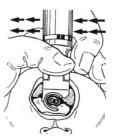

Laryngoscope inserted off to one side.	You see part of the glottis off to one side of the blade.	Gently move the blade back to the midline. Then advance or retreat according to landmarks seen.

Figure 5.30. Common problems associated with intubation

Poor visualization of the glottis also may be caused by not elevating the tongue high enough to bring the glottis into view (Figure 5.31).

Sometimes, pressure applied to the cricoid, which is the cartilage covering the larynx, helps to bring the glottis into view (Figure 5.32).

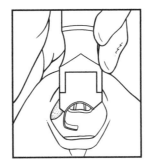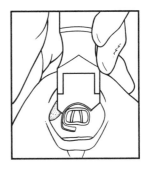

Figure 5.31. Poor visualization of the glottis (left) can be improved by elevating the tongue or depressing the larynx (right)

This is accomplished by using the fourth or fifth finger of the left hand or by asking an assistant to apply the pressure.

Practice intubating a manikin enough times so that you can quickly find the correct landmarks and insert the tube within 20 seconds.

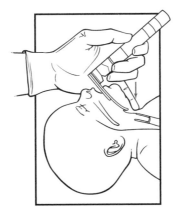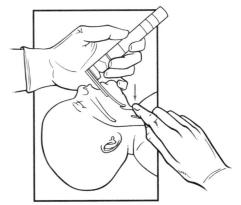

Figure 5.32. Improving visualization with pressure applied to larynx by intubator (left) or by an assistant (right)

You may inadvertently insert the tube into the esophagus instead of the trachea.

An endotracheal tube in the esophagus is worse than having no tube at all, because the tube will obstruct the baby's pharyngeal airway without providing an artificial airway. Therefore,

- Be certain that you visualize the glottis before inserting the tube. Watch the tube enter the glottis between the vocal cords.
- Look carefully for signs of esophageal intubation after the tube has been inserted. Use a CO_2 detector.

If you are concerned that the tube may be in the esophagus, visualize the glottis and tube with a laryngoscope and/or remove the tube, oxygenate the newborn with a bag and mask, and reintroduce the tube.

> **Signs of an endotracheal tube in the esophagus instead of the trachea**
>
> • Poor response to intubation (continued cyanosis, bradycardia, etc)
> • CO_2 detector fails to show presence of expired CO_2
> • No audible breath sounds
> • Air heard entering the stomach
> • Gastric distension may be seen
> • No mist in tube
> • Poor chest movement

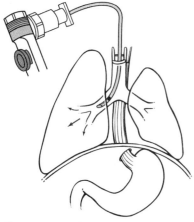

Figure 5.33. Endotracheal tube inserted too far (tip is down the right main bronchus)

You may inadvertently insert the tube too far into the trachea, down the right main bronchus.

If the tube is inserted too far, it usually will pass into the right main bronchus (Figure 5.33).

When you insert the tube, it is important to watch the vocal cord guide on the tube and stop advancing the tube as soon as the vocal cord guide reaches the cords.

Signs of the tube being in the right main bronchus include

• Baby's heart rate or color shows no improvement.

• Breath sounds are heard over the right side of the chest but not the left side.

• Breath sounds are louder on the right side of the chest than on the left side.

If you think the tube may be down the right main bronchus, first check the tip-to-lip measurement to see if the number at the lip is higher than the estimated measurement (Table 5-3). Even if the measurement appears to be correct, if breath sounds remain asymmetric, you should withdraw the tube slightly while you listen over the left side of the chest to hear if the breath sounds improve.

You may encounter other complications (Table 5-4).

Table 5-4. Common complications associated with endotracheal intubation

Complication	Possible Causes	Prevention or Corrective Action to Be Considered
Hypoxia	Taking too long to intubate	Pre-oxygenate with bag and mask. Provide free-flow oxygen during procedure. Halt intubation attempt after 20 seconds.
	Incorrect placement of tube	Reposition tube.
Bradycardia/apnea	Hypoxia Vagal response from laryngoscope or suction catheter	Pre-oxygenate with bag and mask. Provide free-flow oxygen during procedure. Oxygenate after intubation with bag and tube.
Pneumothorax	Overventilation of one lung due to tube in right main bronchus	Place tube correctly.
	Excessive ventilation pressures	Use appropriate ventilating pressures.
Contusions or lacerations of tongue, gums, or airway	Rough handling of laryngoscope or tube Inappropriate "rocking" rather than lifting of laryngoscope	Obtain additional practice/skill.
	Laryngoscope blade too long or too short	Select appropriate equipment.
Perforation of trachea or esophagus	Too vigorous insertion of tube	Handle tube gently.
	Stylet protrudes beyond end of tube	Place stylet properly.
Obstructed endotracheal tube	Kink in tube or tube obstructed with secretions	Try to suction tube with catheter. If unsuccessful, consider replacing tube.
Infection	Introduction of organisms via hands or equipment	Pay careful attention to clean technique.

Key Points

1. A person experienced in endotracheal intubation should be available to assist at every delivery.

2. Indications for endotracheal intubation include the following:
   - To suction trachea in presence of meconium when the newborn is not vigorous
   - To improve efficacy of ventilation after several minutes of bag-and-mask ventilation or ineffective bag-and-mask ventilation
   - To facilitate coordination of chest compressions and ventilation and to maximize the efficiency of each ventilation
   - To administer epinephrine if required to stimulate the heart while intravenous access is being established

3. The laryngoscope is always held in the operator's left hand.

4. The correct-sized laryngoscope blade for a term newborn is No. 1. The correct-sized blade for a preterm newborn is No. 0.

5. Choice of the proper endotracheal tube size is based on weight.

Tube Size (mm) (inside diameter)	Weight (g)	Gestational Age (wks)
2.5	Below 1,000	Below 28
3.0	1,000–2,000	28–34
3.5	2,000–3,000	34–38
3.5–4.0	Above 3,000	Above 38

6. The intubation procedure ideally should be completed within 20 seconds.

7. The steps for intubating a newborn are as follows:
   - Stabilize the newborn's head in the "sniffing" position. Deliver free-flow oxygen during the procedure.
   - Slide the laryngoscope over the right side of the tongue, pushing the tongue to the left side of the mouth, and advancing the blade until the tip lies just beyond the base of the tongue.
   - Lift the blade slightly. Raise the entire blade, not just the tip.
   - Look for landmarks. Vocal cords should appear as vertical stripes on each side of the glottis or as an inverted letter "V".
   - Suction, if necessary, for visualization.
   - Insert the tube into the right side of the mouth with the curve of the tube lying in the horizontal plane.
   - If the cords are closed, wait for them to open. Insert the tip of the endotracheal tube until the vocal cord guide is at the level of the cords.
   - Hold the tube firmly against the baby's palate while removing the laryngoscope. Hold the tube in place while removing the stylet if one was used.

8. Correct placement of the endotracheal tube is indicated by
   - Improved vital signs (heart rate, color, activity)
   - Presence of exhaled CO_2 as determined by a CO_2 detector
   - Breath sounds over both lung fields but decreased or absent over the stomach
   - No gastric distention with ventilation
   - Vapor in the tube during exhalation
   - Chest movement with each breath
   - Tip-to-lip measurement: add 6 to newborn's weight in kilograms
   - Chest x-ray confirmation if the tube is to remain in place past initial resuscitation
   - Direct visualization of the tube passing between the vocal cords

Lesson 5 Review

(The answers follow.)

1. A newborn with meconium and depressed respirations (will) (will not) require suctioning by endotracheal intubation before positive-pressure ventilation is administered.

2. A newborn receiving ventilation by bag and mask is not improving after 2 minutes of apparently good technique. The heart rate is not rising and there is poor chest movement. Endotracheal intubation (should) (should not) be considered.

3. For babies weighing less than 1,000 g, the inside size of the endotracheal tube should be _____ mm.

4. The blade of a laryngoscope for preterm newborns should be No. _____. The blade for term newborns should be No. _____.

5. Which illustration shows the view of the oral cavity that you should see if you have the laryngoscope correctly placed for intubation?

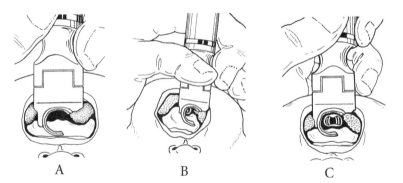

      A   B   C

6. Both right- and left-handed people should hold the laryngoscope in their _____ hand.

7. You should try to take no longer than _____ seconds to complete endotracheal intubation.

8. If you have not completed endotracheal intubation within the time limit in Question 7, what should you do?

_____

Lesson 5 Review—*continued*

(The answers follow.)

9. Which illustration shows the correct way to lift the tongue out of the way to expose the pharyngeal area?

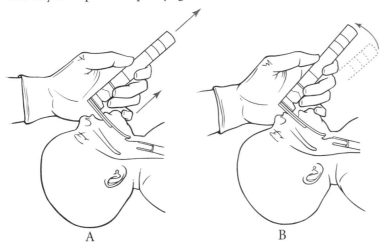

A   B

10. You have the glottis in view, but the vocal cords are closed. You (should) (should not) wait until they are open to insert the tube.

11. How far should the endotracheal tube be inserted into the baby's trachea? _____

12. You have inserted an endotracheal tube and are giving positive-pressure ventilation through it. When you check with a stethoscope, you hear breath sounds on both sides of the baby's chest, with equal intensity on each side and no air entering the stomach. The tube (is) (is not) correctly placed.

13. Which x-ray shows the correct placement of an endotracheal tube?

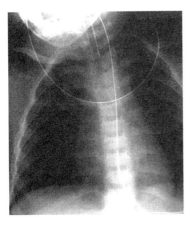
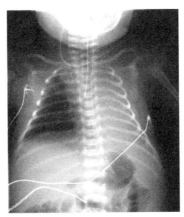

A   B

14. You have inserted an endotracheal tube and are giving positive-pressure ventilation through it. When you check with a stethoscope, you hear no breath sounds over either side of the chest and you hear air entering the stomach. The tube is placed in the (esophagus) (trachea).

15. If the tube is in the esophagus, it must be removed, the newborn given _____ by bag and mask, and the tube reinserted correctly.

16. You have inserted an endotracheal tube and are giving positive-pressure ventilation through it. When you check with a stethoscope, you hear breath sounds over the right side of the chest, but not the left. When you check the tip-to-lip measurement, it is higher than expected. You should (withdraw) (insert) the tube slightly and listen with the stethoscope again.

Answers to Questions

1. A newborn with meconium and depressed respirations **will** require suctioning by endotracheal intubation before positive-pressure ventilation is administered.

2. Endotracheal intubation **should** be considered for a newborn who is not improving, despite good technique.

3. For babies weighing less than 1,000 g, the inside size of the endotracheal tube should be **2.5** mm.

4. The blade of a laryngoscope should be No. **0** for preterm newborns and No. **1** for term newborns.

5. Illustration **C** shows the correct view for intubation.

6. Both right- and left-handed people should hold the laryngoscope in their **left** hand.

7. The goal should be to insert an endotracheal tube and connect it to a bag within **20 seconds.**

8. If you have not completed endotracheal intubation within 20 seconds, you should **remove the laryngoscope, ventilate with bag and mask, and then try again.**

9. Illustration **A** is correct.

10. You **should** wait until the vocal cords are open to insert the tube.

11. You should insert the tube **to the level of the vocal cord guide.**

12. The tube **is** correctly placed.

13. X-ray **A** shows correct placement of an endotracheal tube.

14. The tube is placed in the **esophagus.**

15. The newborn should be given **ventilation** by bag and mask. The tube then should be reinserted correctly.

16. You should **withdraw** the tube slightly and listen with the stethoscope again.

Performance Checklist

Lesson 5 — Endotracheal Intubation

Instructor: The learner should be instructed to talk through the procedure as it is demonstrated. Judge the performance of each step and check (✓) the box when the action is completed correctly. If done incorrectly, circle the box so that you can discuss that step later. You will need to provide information at several points concerning the condition of the baby.

Learner: To successfully complete this checklist, you should be able to perform all the steps and make all the correct decisions in the procedure. You should talk through the procedure as you perform it.

Equipment and Supplies

Intubation manikin

Radiant warmer or tabletop to simulate warmer

Gloves (or may be implied)

Stethoscope

Shoulder roll

Laryngoscope with fresh batteries and functioning light source

Blade, No. 1 (term) for use with manikin or No. 0, if appropriate

Endotracheal tubes, 2.5, 3.0, 3.5, 4.0 mm

Stylet (optional)

Tape or endotracheal tube securing device

Scissors (optional)

Mechanical suction device (or may be implied) with 10F or larger suction catheter

Self-inflating bag

or

Flow-inflating bag with pressure manometer and oxygen source

or

T-piece resuscitator with oxygen source

Method to administer free-flow oxygen (oxygen mask, oxygen tubing, or flow-inflating bag and mask) (Oxygen may be simulated.)

Flowmeter (or may simulate this)

Masks (term and preterm sizes)

Meconium aspirator

CO_2 detector

Clock with second hand

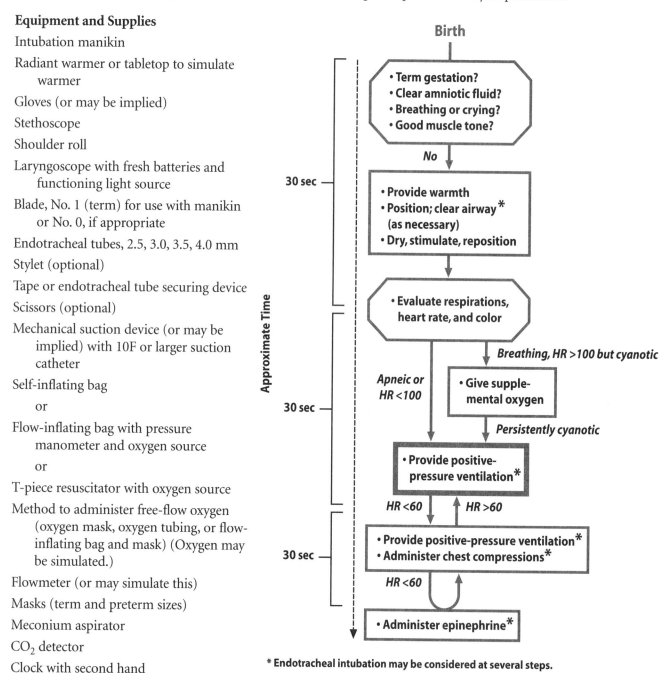

* Endotracheal intubation may be considered at several steps.

Performance Checklist

Lesson 5 — Endotracheal Intubation

Name _____ Instructor _____ Date _____

This performance checklist can be completed by learners who will be responsible for intubating and/or by those who will be assisting with intubation. If only one learner is being evaluated, the instructor may take the role of the other person.

Instructor's questions are in quotes. Learner's questions and correct responses are in bold type. Instructor should check boxes as the learner answers correctly.

Section A — Preparing for Intubation

"A full-term baby is about to be born. There have been severe fetal heart rate decelerations and there is meconium in the amniotic fluid. How would you prepare for this situation and assist with the activity?"

Endotracheal Tube

☐ **Selects correct-sized tube**

☐ **Cuts tube at 13 or 15 cm and replaces connector, securing a tight fit (optional)**

☐ **Inserts stylet (optional)**

  ☐ **Stylet tip is *within* tip of tube**

  ☐ **Secures stylet**

Laryngoscope

☐ **Selects appropriate-sized blade**

☐ **Attaches blade to laryngoscope and checks light — replaces batteries or bulb if necessary**

Additional Equipment

☐ **Obtains**
  • **Oxygen tubing and source**
  • **Suction equipment**

☐ **Obtains bag and mask**

  ☐ **Checks bag for function**

  ☐ **Prepares bag to give 90% to 100% oxygen**

  ☐ **Selects appropriate-sized mask**

☐ **Obtains meconium aspiration device**

☐ **Obtains CO_2 detection device**

☐ **Cuts strips of tape or prepares endotracheal tube securing device**

Section B — Performing or Assisting With Endotracheal Intubation

If you will be intubating rather than assisting, you will be asked to do this procedure twice. The first time, you should "talk through" the procedure, describing each action or observation made. This is necessary because your instructor is unable to view all aspects of the procedure directly.

The second time through, you do not need to describe what you are doing. Instead, work as quickly and efficiently as possible to complete the procedure within 20 seconds—from laryngoscope placement through tube insertion.

"The baby has just been born, and her skin is covered with meconium. She is placed under a radiant warmer and is limp. Demonstrate what you would do."

Performs Intubation   **Assists**

- [ ] Correctly positions manikin   [ ]
- [ ] Uses/provides free-flow oxygen   [ ]
- [ ] Provides suction when requested   [ ]
- [ ] Inserts blade into mouth, holding laryngoscope correctly
- [ ] Inserts blade just beyond tongue and lifts using correct motion
- [ ] Applies laryngeal pressure correctly when asked   [ ]
- [ ] Identifies landmarks seen
- [ ] Based on landmarks seen, takes corrective action if applicable
- [ ] Obtains unobstructed view of glottis
- [ ] Inserts tube into trachea
- [ ] Removes laryngoscope (and stylet if used) while firmly holding tube in place
- [ ] Connects (or assists with) meconium aspirator   [ ]
- [ ] Withdraws tube while applying suction
- [ ] Performs entire procedure within 20 seconds

"Assume that no further meconium is recovered during suctioning. The baby is limp and fails to resume spontaneous respirations following stimulation and several minutes of bag-and-mask ventilation. Although the baby is pink and has a heart rate greater than 100 bpm, you have decided to reinsert the endotracheal tube for continued positive-pressure ventilation."

Performs Intubation   Assists

☐ Administers positive-pressure ventilation with bag and mask   ☐

☐ Correctly positions manikin   ☐

☐ Uses/provides free-flow oxygen   ☐

☐ Provides suction when requested   ☐

☐ Inserts blade into mouth, holding laryngoscope correctly

☐ Inserts blade just beyond tongue and lifts using correct motion

☐ Applies laryngeal pressure correctly when asked   ☐

☐ Identifies landmarks seen

☐ Based on landmarks seen, takes corrective action if applicable

☐ Obtains unobstructed view of glottis

☐ Inserts tube, aligning vocal cord guide with vocal cords

☐ Removes laryngoscope (and stylet if used) while firmly holding tube so that tube position does not change

☐ Removes mask from bag and attaches to endotracheal tube and inflates lungs   ☐

☐ Consumes/notes no more than 20 seconds from blade insertion through correct tube placement   ☐

Provides Initial Confirmation of Placement

☐ Correctly states steps for confirming placement   ☐

☐ Notes improving vital signs

☐ Attaches CO_2 detection device and observes change in color

☐ Auscultates equal breath sounds over both lung fields, but not over stomach

☐ Does not observe increasing gastric distension

☐ Observes vapor condensing on inside of tube during exhalation

☐ Notes symmetrical movement of chest

"You have connected the resuscitation bag to the tube and resumed positive-pressure ventilation. However, the baby is cyanotic and the heart rate is 80 bpm."

☐ **Assesses need for corrective action and performs the necessary steps if tube is in esophagus or one of the bronchi**

    ☐ **Repeats confirmation steps**

    ☐ **Correctly assesses tip-to-lip measurement**

    ☐ **Reinserts laryngoscope and visualizes placement of stripe at vocal cords**

        and/or

    ☐ **Removes endotracheal tube, ventilates with bag and mask, and repeats intubation**

"The baby's color has improved and the heart rate is now greater than 100 bpm. However, the baby remains apneic and you have decided to leave the tube in place during transfer to post-resuscitation care."

Takes Final Steps

    ☐ **States centimeter marking at level of upper lip**

    ☐ **Secures tube while maintaining proper position**
        (technique will depend on specific method used in learner's hospital)

    ☐ **Shortens tube if more than 4 cm extends from lips**

Overall Assessment

    ☐ **Gently handles baby, laryngoscope, and endotracheal tube to prevent trauma**

    ☐ **Limits attempts to 20 seconds**

Appendix
Use of a Laryngeal Mask Airway

In this Appendix, you will learn
- What a laryngeal mask airway is
- When to consider using a laryngeal mask airway for positive-pressure ventilation
- How to place a laryngeal mask airway

The following case is an example of how a laryngeal mask airway can be used to provide positive-pressure ventilation during neonatal resuscitation. As you read the case, imagine yourself as part of the resuscitation team. The details of this procedure will be described in the remainder of this Appendix.

Case 5.
Difficult intubation

A baby is delivered at term after a labor complicated by fetal decelerations. The fluid is clear, without meconium staining. The baby is brought to the radiant warmer limp, blue, and apneic. The initial steps of resuscitation are performed and positive-pressure ventilation is initiated with a bag-and-mask device and supplemental oxygen, but the team cannot achieve effective ventilation, despite appropriate adjustments. The resuscitation team unsuccessfully attempts to place an endotracheal tube using direct laryngoscopy. The team leader notes that the baby has a relatively large tongue, small jaw, and facial features consistent with Down syndrome. The infant remains limp, blue, and apneic.

One team member rapidly places a laryngeal mask airway, attaches a resuscitation bag, and achieves effective positive-pressure ventilation, resulting in an increasing heart rate and good breath sounds. The baby's color improves, and she begins to show spontaneous respirations. As she becomes more responsive, the laryngeal mask airway is removed and she is transferred to the neonatal intensive care unit for further evaluation and post-resuscitative care.

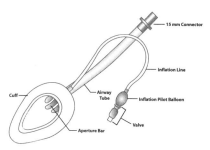

Figure 5.34. Size-1 neonatal laryngeal mask airway

What is a laryngeal mask airway?

The laryngeal mask airway is an airway device that can be used to provide positive-pressure ventilation. The size-1 neonatal device (Figure 5.34) is a soft elliptical mask with an inflatable rim attached to a flexible airway tube. The device is inserted into the baby's mouth with your index finger and guided along the baby's hard palate until the tip nearly reaches the esophagus. No instruments are used. Once the mask is fully inserted, the rim is inflated. The inflated mask covers the laryngeal opening and the rim conforms to the contours of the hypopharynx occluding the esophagus with a low-pressure seal. The airway tube has a standard 15-mm adaptor that is attached to either a resuscitation bag or ventilator. A pilot balloon attached to the rim is used to monitor the mask's inflation. Both reusable and disposable versions are commercially available.

How does a laryngeal mask airway work?

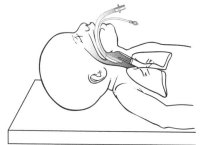

Figure 5.35. Laryngeal mask airway in place over the laryngeal opening

The larynx is a firm structure that forms the opening of the trachea into the anterior pharynx. The distal end of the device is a soft mask that functions like a cap that fits over the larynx. The mask has a donut-shaped rim (cuff) that can be inflated to make a seal over the larynx (Figure 5.35). The mask has bars across the middle that prevent the epiglottis from becoming trapped within the airway tube. (See "aperture bar" in Figure 5.34.) After the mask has been placed over the larynx, the cuff is inflated, thus providing a seal. When positive pressure is applied to the airway tube, the pressure is transmitted through the airway tube and the mask, into the baby's trachea.

When should you consider using a laryngeal mask airway?

Laryngeal mask airways may be useful in situations when positive pressure with a face mask fails to achieve effective ventilation, and attempts at endotracheal intubation have been either unfeasible or unsuccessful. When you "can't ventilate and can't intubate," the device may provide a successful rescue airway.

For example, a laryngeal mask airway may be helpful when an infant presents with the following:

- Congenital anomalies involving the mouth, lip, or palate, when achieving a good seal with a bag and mask is difficult
- Anomalies of the mouth, tongue, pharynx, or neck, when there is difficulty visualizing the larynx with a laryngoscope
- A very small mandible or relatively large tongue, such as with Robin syndrome and Down syndrome

The laryngeal mask airway also may be helpful when

- Positive-pressure ventilation provided by bag and mask or T-piece resuscitator is ineffective, and attempts at intubation are not feasible or are unsuccessful.

The laryngeal mask airway does not require a firm seal against the face. Furthermore, unlike a firm face mask, the flexible laryngeal mask bypasses the tongue, allowing more effective ventilation of the lungs than with a face mask. In addition, no instrument is needed to visualize the larynx to place the device. It is placed "blindly" by using the operator's finger to guide it into place without any instruments. Although a laryngeal mask airway does not provide as tight a seal in the airway as an endotracheal tube, it can provide an acceptable alternative in some cases.

The laryngeal mask airway is used by anesthesiologists for ventilating patients with normal lungs during anesthesia in many hospital operating rooms.

What are the limitations of the laryngeal mask airway?

- The device cannot be used to suction meconium from the airway.
- If you need to use high ventilation pressures, air may leak through an insufficient seal between the larynx and the mask, resulting in insufficient pressure to inflate the lungs and causing gastric distention.
- There is insufficient evidence to recommend the laryngeal mask when chest compressions are required. However, if an endotracheal tube cannot be placed successfully and chest compressions are required, it is reasonable to attempt compressions with the device in place.
- There is insufficient evidence to recommend the laryngeal mask when intratracheal medications are required. Intratracheal medications may leak between the mask and larynx, into the esophagus and, therefore, not enter the lung.
- There is insufficient evidence to recommend the laryngeal mask for prolonged assisted ventilation in newborns.

Are there different sizes of laryngeal mask airways?

The size-1 device is the only size appropriate for newborns. It has been used primarily in term and near-term infants weighing >2,500 g. There has been limited experience using the laryngeal mask in infants between 1,500 and 2,500 g. It is probably too large for babies with a birth weight <1,500 g.

How do you place the laryngeal mask airway?

The following instructions apply to the disposable device. If you are using the reusable laryngeal mask, refer to the manufacturer's instructions for proper cleaning and maintenance procedures.

Prepare the laryngeal mask airway.

1. Wear gloves and follow standard precautions.

2. Remove the size-1 device from the sterile package and use clean technique.

3. Quickly inspect the device to ensure that the mask, midline aperture bars, airway tube, 15-mm connector, and pilot balloon are intact.

4. Attach the included syringe to the pilot balloon valve port and test the mask by inflating it with 4 mL of air. Using the attached syringe, remove the air from the mask.

Get ready to insert the laryngeal mask airway.

5. Stand at the infant's head and position the head in the "sniffing" position as you would for endotracheal intubation.

6. Hold the device like a pen, with your index finger placed at the junction of the cuff and the tube (Figure 5.36). The bars in the middle of the mask opening must be facing forward. The flat part of the mask has no bars or openings and it will be facing the baby's palate.

7. Some clinicians advise lubricating the back of the laryngeal mask with water-soluble lubricant. If you do so, be careful to keep the lubricant away from the apertures on the front side, inside the mask.

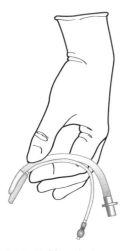

Figure 5.36. Holding the laryngeal mask airway prior to insertion

Insert the laryngeal mask airway.

8. Gently open the baby's mouth and press the leading tip of the mask against the baby's hard palate (Figure 5.37A).

9. Flatten the tip of the mask against the baby's palate with your index finger. Ensure that the tip of the mask remains flat and does not curl backward on itself.

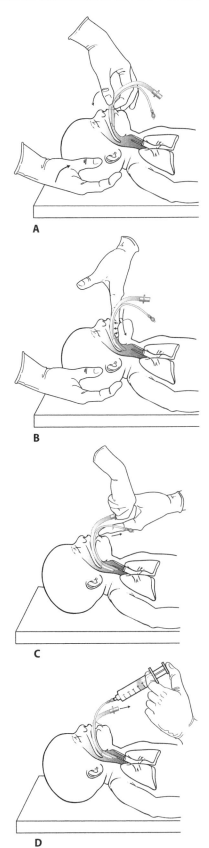

10. Using your index finger, gently guide the device along the contours of the baby's hard palate toward the back of the throat (Figure 5.37B). **Do not use force.** Use a smooth movement to guide the mask past the tongue and into the hypopharynx until you feel resistance.

Set the laryngeal mask airway in place.

11. Before removing your finger, use your other hand to hold the airway tube in place (Figure 5.37C). This prevents the device from being pulled out of place when your finger is removed. At this point, the tip of the mask should be resting near the entrance to the esophagus (upper esophageal sphincter).

12. Inflate the mask with 2 to 4 mL of air (Figure 5.37D). The cuff should be inflated with only enough air to achieve a seal. Do not hold the airway tube when you inflate the mask. You may note that the device moves slightly outward when it is inflated. This is normal. **Never inflate the cuff of the size-1 laryngeal mask airway with more than 4 mL of air.**

Figure 5.37. Inserting and securing the laryngeal mask airway. Although not shown in the figures, the cuff should be inserted deflated and then be inflated after insertion

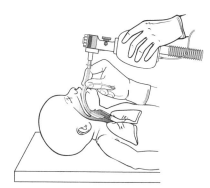

Figure 5.38. Providing positive-pressure ventilation using a laryngeal mask airway

Secure and ventilate through the laryngeal mask airway.

13. Attach your resuscitation bag to the 15-mm adaptor on the device and begin positive-pressure ventilation (Figure 5.38).

14. Confirm proper placement by assessing rising heart rate, chest wall movement, and audible breath sounds with a stethoscope. An end-tidal carbon dioxide (CO_2) monitor may be used to confirm adequate gas exchange.

15. Secure the tube with tape, as you would for an endotracheal tube.

How do you know that the laryngeal mask airway is properly placed?

If the device is properly placed, you should notice a prompt increase in the baby's heart rate, equal breath sounds when you listen with a stethoscope, and chest wall movement, similar to what you would expect with a properly placed endotracheal tube. If you place a colorimetric CO_2 monitor on the adaptor, you should note a rapid color change indicating expired CO_2. You should not hear a large leak of air coming from the baby's mouth or see a growing bulge in the baby's neck.

What are the possible complications that may occur with the laryngeal mask airway?

The device may cause soft-tissue trauma, laryngospasm, or gastric air distension from air leaking around the mask. Prolonged use over hours or days has been infrequently associated with oropharyngeal nerve damage or lingual edema.

When should you remove the laryngeal mask airway?

The laryngeal mask airway can be removed when the baby establishes effective spontaneous respirations or when an endotracheal tube can be inserted successfully. Babies can breathe spontaneously through the device. If necessary, the laryngeal mask airway can be attached to a ventilator or continuous positive airway pressure (CPAP) device during transport to the neonatal intensive care unit, but long-term use for ventilation of newborns has not been investigated.

Medications

In Lesson 6 you will learn

- **What medications to give during resuscitation**
- **When to give medications during resuscitation**
- **Where to give medications during resuscitation**
- **How to insert an umbilical venous catheter**
- **How to administer epinephrine**
- **When and how to administer fluids intravenously to expand blood volume during a resuscitation**

The following case is an example of how medications may be used during an extensive resuscitation. As you read the case, imagine yourself as part of the resuscitation team. The details of medications administration are described in the remainder of the lesson.

Case 6.
Resuscitation with positive-pressure ventilation, chest compressions, and medications

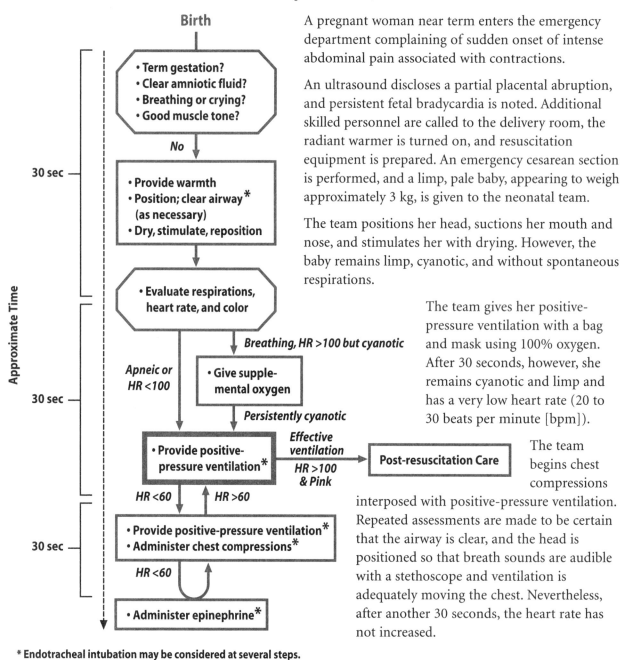

A pregnant woman near term enters the emergency department complaining of sudden onset of intense abdominal pain associated with contractions.

An ultrasound discloses a partial placental abruption, and persistent fetal bradycardia is noted. Additional skilled personnel are called to the delivery room, the radiant warmer is turned on, and resuscitation equipment is prepared. An emergency cesarean section is performed, and a limp, pale baby, appearing to weigh approximately 3 kg, is given to the neonatal team.

The team positions her head, suctions her mouth and nose, and stimulates her with drying. However, the baby remains limp, cyanotic, and without spontaneous respirations.

The team gives her positive-pressure ventilation with a bag and mask using 100% oxygen. After 30 seconds, however, she remains cyanotic and limp and has a very low heart rate (20 to 30 beats per minute [bpm]).

The team begins chest compressions interposed with positive-pressure ventilation. Repeated assessments are made to be certain that the airway is clear, and the head is positioned so that breath sounds are audible with a stethoscope and ventilation is adequately moving the chest. Nevertheless, after another 30 seconds, the heart rate has not increased.

* Endotracheal intubation may be considered at several steps.

The team rapidly intubates the trachea to ensure effective ventilation and begins to insert an umbilical venous catheter. The heart rate is now undetectable, so 1.5 mL of 1:10,000 epinephrine is instilled into the endotracheal tube while umbilical venous access is being established. The heart rate is checked every 30 seconds as coordinated chest compressions and positive-pressure ventilation continue. The heart rate remains undetectable.

By 3 minutes of age, placement of an umbilical venous catheter is underway and, soon after, a dose of 0.6 mL of epinephrine is given into the catheter, followed by a normal saline flush. The heart rate is now audible with a stethoscope, but remains less than 60 bpm. Because the baby has persistent bradycardia and a history of possible blood loss, 30 mL of normal saline is given into the umbilical catheter. The heart rate gradually increases.

By 7 minutes after birth, the baby makes an initial gasp. Chest compressions are stopped when the heart rate rises above 60 bpm. Assisted ventilation continues with supplemental oxygen and the heart rate rises above 100 bpm. The baby's color begins to improve, and she begins to have spontaneous respirations.

She is transferred to the nursery for post-resuscitation care, with assisted ventilation still underway.

If resuscitation steps are implemented in a skillful and timely manner, more than 99% of newborns requiring resuscitation will improve without the need for medications. Before administering medications, you should have checked the effectiveness of ventilation several times, ensuring good chest movement and audible bilateral breath sounds with each breath, and that you are using 100% oxygen for positive-pressure ventilation. As part of this assessment, you may have inserted an endotracheal tube to ensure a good airway and effective coordination of chest compressions and positive-pressure ventilation.

 If the heart rate remains below 60 bpm, despite administration of ventilation and chest compressions, your first action is to ensure that ventilation and compressions are being given optimally and that you are using 100% oxygen.

Despite good ventilation of the lungs with positive-pressure ventilation and improved cardiac output from chest compressions, a small number of newborns (fewer than 2 per 1,000 births) will still have a heart rate below 60 bpm. The heart muscle of these babies may have been deprived of oxygen for so long that it will not contract effectively, despite now being perfused with oxygenated blood. These babies may benefit from receiving epinephrine to stimulate the heart. If there has been acute blood loss, they may benefit from volume replacement.

What will this lesson cover?

This lesson will teach you when to give *epinephrine,* how to establish a route by which to give it, and how to determine dosage.

The lesson also will discuss *volume expansion* for babies in shock from acute blood loss.

Administration of naloxone, a narcotic antagonist given to babies who have depressed respirations from maternal narcotics, is not necessary during the acute phases of resuscitation and will be discussed in Lesson 7. Sodium bicarbonate may be used to treat metabolic acidosis, and vasopressors, such as dopamine, may be used for hypotension or poor cardiac output, but these are administered more often in the post-resuscitative period and are discussed in Lesson 7. Other drugs, such as atropine and calcium, are sometimes used during special resuscitation circumstances, but are not indicated during the acute phase of neonatal resuscitation.

If any medications are required, you will learn that the most reliable route of administration is the intravenous route. Therefore, as soon as you suspect that medications may be needed, you should call for help. While a minimum of 2 people are required to administer coordinated positive-pressure ventilation and chest compressions, a third and perhaps fourth person will be required to begin establishment of an intravenous line.

How do you establish intravenous access during resuscitation of a newborn?

The umbilical vein
The umbilical vein is the most quickly accessible direct intravenous route in the newborn. If the use of epinephrine is anticipated because of unresponsiveness of the baby to the earlier steps of resuscitation, one member of the resuscitation team should begin work on placing an umbilical venous catheter, while others continue the other steps of resuscitation.

- Clean the cord with an antiseptic solution. Place a loose tie of umbilical tape around the base of the cord. This tie can be tightened if there is excessive bleeding after you cut the cord.

- Pre-fill a 3.5F or 5F umbilical catheter with normal saline using a 3-mL syringe connected to a stopcock. The catheter should have a single end-hole. Close the stopcock to the catheter to prevent fluid loss and air entry.

- Using sterile technique, cut the cord with a scalpel below the clamp that had been placed at birth and about 1 to 2 cm from the skin line (Figure 6.1). Make the cut perpendicular to the umbilical cord, rather than at an angle.

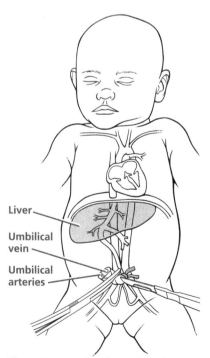

Liver

Umbilical vein

Umbilical arteries

Figure 6.1. Cutting the umbilical stump in preparation for inserting umbilical catheter

- The umbilical vein will be seen as a large, thin-walled structure, usually at the 11- to 12-o'clock position. The 2 umbilical arteries have thicker walls and usually lie close together somewhere in the 4- and 8-o'clock positions. However, the arteries coil within the cord. Therefore, the longer the cord stump below your cut, the greater the likelihood that the vessels will not lie in the positions described.

- Insert the catheter into the umbilical vein (Figure 6.2). (Also see color Figures E-1 and E-2 in the center of the book.) The course of the vein will be up, toward the heart, so this is the direction you should point the catheter. Continue inserting the catheter 2 to 4 cm (less in preterm babies) until you get free flow of blood when you open the stopcock to the syringe and gently aspirate. For emergency use during resuscitation, the tip of the catheter should be located only a short distance into the vein—only to the point at which blood is first able to be aspirated. If the catheter is inserted farther, there is risk of infusing most of the solution directly into the liver and possibly causing damage.

- Inject the appropriate dose of epinephrine or volume expander (see pages 6-6 through 6-10), followed by 0.5 to 1 mL of normal saline to clear the drug from the catheter into the baby.

- Once the baby has been fully resuscitated, either suture the catheter in place or remove the catheter, tighten the cord tie, and complete the knot to prevent bleeding from the umbilical stump. Do not advance the catheter once the sterile field has been violated.

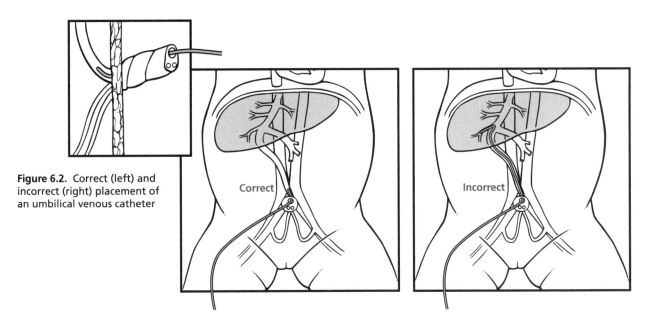

Figure 6.2. Correct (left) and incorrect (right) placement of an umbilical venous catheter

Correct

Incorrect

Are there alternatives to intravenous access for administration of medications during resuscitation of a newborn?

The endotracheal tube

Epinephrine given into the endotracheal tube may be absorbed by the lungs and enter blood that drains directly into the heart. Although this may be the fastest way to give epinephrine in an intubated baby, the process of absorption by the lungs makes the response time slower and more unpredictable than if epinephrine is given directly into the blood. Research in animal models suggests that the standard intravenous dose is ineffective if given endotracheally. There is some evidence that giving a higher dose can compensate for the delayed absorption from the lungs; however, no studies have confirmed the efficacy or safety of this practice. Nevertheless, since the endotracheal route is the most readily accessible, some clinicians believe that an endotracheal dose should be considered while the intravenous route is being established. If endotracheal epinephrine is given, a larger dose will be needed and, therefore, a larger syringe will be necessary. The large syringe should be clearly labeled "For Endotracheal Use Only," to avoid inadvertently giving the higher dose intravenously. While this program will mention the endotracheal technique, the intravascular route is recommended as the best choice.

Intraosseous access

When resuscitating a newborn in the hospital setting, the umbilical vein is clearly the most readily available vascular access. However, in the outpatient setting, where health care providers have limited experience with umbilical catheterization and may have had more experience with placement of intraosseous lines, this may be a preferable alternative for vascular access. However, there are limited data evaluating the use of intraosseous lines in newborns, and the intraosseous technique will not be taught in this program.

What is epinephrine and when should you give it?

Epinephrine hydrochloride (sometimes referred to as adrenaline chloride) is a cardiac stimulant. Epinephrine increases the strength and rate of cardiac contractions and causes peripheral vasoconstriction, which may increase blood flow through the coronary arteries and to the brain.

 Epinephrine is indicated when the heart rate remains below 60 bpm after you have given 30 seconds of effective assisted ventilation and another 30 seconds of coordinated chest compressions and ventilation.

Epinephrine is not indicated before you have established adequate ventilation because

- Time spent administering epinephrine is better spent on establishing effective ventilation and oxygenation.
- Epinephrine will increase workload and oxygen consumption of the heart muscle, which, in the absence of available oxygen, may cause myocardial damage.

How should you prepare epinephrine and how much should you give?

Although epinephrine is available in both 1:1,000 and 1:10,000 concentrations, the 1:10,000 concentration is recommended for newborns, eliminating the need for dilution.

Epinephrine should be given intravenously, although administration may be delayed by the time required to establish intravenous access. The endotracheal route is usually quicker, but this route results in lower and unpredictable blood levels that may not be effective. Some clinicians may choose to give a dose of endotracheal epinephrine while the umbilical venous line is being placed.

The recommended intravenous dose in newborns is 0.1 to 0.3 mL/kg of a 1:10,000 solution (equal to 0.01 to 0.03 mg/kg). You will need to estimate the baby's weight after birth.

In the past, higher intravenous doses had been suggested for adults and older children when they did not respond to a lower dose. However, there is no evidence that this results in a better outcome and there is some evidence that higher doses in babies may result in brain and heart damage.

Animal and adult human studies demonstrate that, when given via the trachea, significantly higher doses of epinephrine than previously recommended are required to show a positive effect. If you decide to give a dose endotracheally while intravenous access is being obtained, consider giving a higher dose (0.3 to 1 mL/kg, or 0.03 to 0.1 mg/kg) by this route only. However, the safety of these higher tracheal doses has not been studied. *Do not give high doses intravenously.*

When giving epinephrine by endotracheal tube, be sure to give the drug directly into the tube, being careful not to leave it deposited in the endotracheal tube connector or along the walls of the tube. Some people prefer to use a catheter to give the drug deeply into the tube. Because you will need to give a higher dose endotracheally, you will be giving a relatively large volume of fluid into the endotracheal tube (up to 1 mL/kg). You should follow the drug with several positive-pressure breaths to distribute the drug throughout the lungs for absorption.

When the drug is given intravenously through a catheter, you should follow the drug with a 0.5- to 1-mL flush of normal saline to be sure that the drug has reached the blood.

Recommended concentration = 1:10,000

Recommended route = Intravenously (consider endotracheal route while intravenous access being obtained)

Recommended dose = 0.1 to 0.3 mL/kg of 1:10,000 solution (consider 0.3 to 1 mL/kg if giving endotracheally)

Recommended preparation = 1:10,000 solution in 1-mL syringe (or larger syringe if giving endotracheally)

Recommended rate of administration = *Rapidly*—as quickly as possible

Review

(The answers are in the preceding section and at the end of the lesson.)

1. Fewer than _____ babies per 1,000 births will need epinephrine to stimulate their hearts.

2. As soon as you suspect that medications may be needed during a resuscitation, one member of the team should begin to insert an _____ to deliver the drug(s).

3. Effective ventilation and coordinated chest compressions have been performed for 30 seconds and the baby's heart rate is less than 60 beats per minute. You should now give _____ while continuing chest compressions and _____.

4. What is the problem with administering epinephrine through an endotracheal tube?_____.

5. You should follow an intravenous dose of epinephrine with a flush of _____ to ensure that most of the drug is delivered to the baby and not left in the catheter.

6. Epinephrine (increases) (decreases) the strength of cardiac contractions and (increases) (decreases) the rate of cardiac contractions.

7. The recommended concentration of epinephrine for newborns is (1:1,000) (1:10,000).

8. The recommended dose of epinephrine for newborns is ___ to ___ mL/kg, if given intravenously, and ___ to ___ mL/kg, if given intratracheally, of a 1:10,000 solution.

9. Epinephrine should be given (slowly) (as quickly as possible).

What should you expect to happen after giving epinephrine?

Check the baby's heart rate 30 seconds after administering epinephrine. As you continue positive-pressure ventilation and chest compressions, the heart rate should increase to more than 60 bpm within 30 seconds after you give epinephrine.

If this does not happen, you can repeat the dose every 3 to 5 minutes. However, any repeat doses should be given intravenously if possible. In addition, ensure that

- There is good air exchange as evidenced by adequate chest movement and presence of bilateral breath sounds.
- Chest compressions are given to a depth of one third the diameter of the chest and are well coordinated with ventilations.

Strongly consider placement of an endotracheal tube, if one has not already been inserted. Once in place, ensure that the tube has remained in the trachea during cardiopulmonary resuscitation activities.

If the baby is pale, there is evidence of blood loss, and there is poor response to resuscitation, you will want to consider the possibility of volume loss. Treatment of hypovolemia is covered next.

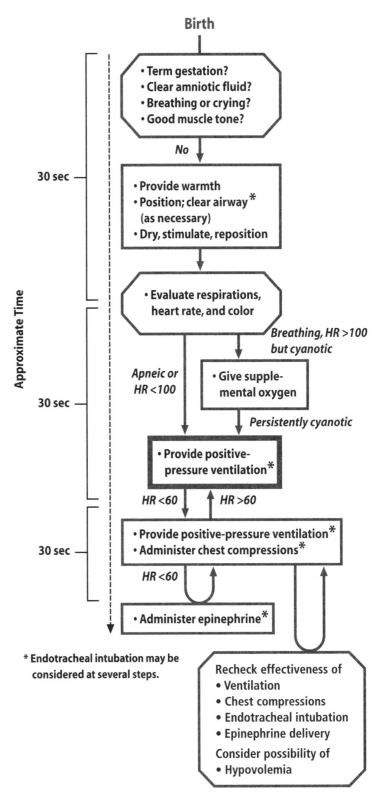

What should you do if the baby is in shock, there is evidence of blood loss, and the baby is responding poorly to resuscitation?

If there has been a placental abruption, a placenta previa, or blood loss from the umbilical cord, the baby may be in hypovolemic shock. In some cases, the baby may have lost blood into the maternal circulation and there will be signs of shock with no obvious evidence of blood loss.

Babies in shock appear pale, have delayed capillary refill, and have weak pulses. They may have a persistently low heart rate, and circulatory status often does not improve in response to effective ventilation, chest compressions, and epinephrine.

 If the baby appears to be in shock and is not responding to resuscitation, administration of a volume expander may be indicated.

What can you give to expand blood volume? How much should you give? How can you give it?

The recommended solution for acutely treating hypovolemia is an isotonic crystalloid solution. Acceptable solutions include

- 0.9% NaCl ("Normal saline").
- Ringer's lactate.
- O Rh-negative packed red blood cells should be considered as part of the volume replacement when severe fetal anemia is documented or expected. If timely diagnosis permits, the donor unit can be cross matched to the mother who would be the source of any problematic antibody. Otherwise, emergency release O Rh-negative packed cells may be necessary.

Recommended solution = Normal saline

The initial dose is 10 mL/kg. However, if the baby shows minimal improvement after the first dose, you may need to give another dose of 10 mL/kg. In unusual cases of large blood loss, additional doses might be considered.

Recommended dose = 10 mL/kg

A volume expander must be given into the vascular system. The umbilical vein is usually the most accessible vein in a newborn, although other routes (eg, intraosseous) can be used.

Recommended route = Umbilical vein

If hypovolemia is suspected, fill a large syringe with normal saline or other volume expander while others on the team continue resuscitation.

Acute hypovolemia, resulting in a need for resuscitation, should be corrected fairly quickly, although some clinicians are concerned that rapid administration in a newborn may result in intracranial hemorrhage, particularly in preterm infants. No clinical trials have been conducted to define an optimum rate, but a steady infusion rate over 5 to 10 minutes is reasonable.

Recommended rate of administration = Over 5–10 minutes

Review

(The answers are in the preceding section and at the end of the lesson.)

10. What should you do approximately 30 seconds after giving epinephrine?

11. If the baby's heart rate remains below 60 beats per minute, you can repeat the dose of epinephrine every _____ to _____ minutes.

12. If the baby's heart rate remains below 60 beats per minute after you have given epinephrine, you also should check to make sure that ventilation is producing adequate lung inflation, and that

    _____ are

    being done correctly.

13. If the baby appears to be in shock, there is evidence of blood loss, and resuscitation is not resulting in improvement, you should consider giving _____ mL/kg of _____

    by _____.

What should you do if there is still no improvement?

If the baby has been severely compromised but all resuscitation efforts have gone smoothly, you should have reached the point of giving epinephrine relatively quickly. Approximately 30 seconds each should be required for a trial of each of the following 4 steps of resuscitation (additional time may be required to be certain that each step is being performed optimally):

- Assessment and initial steps
- Positive-pressure ventilation
- Positive-pressure ventilation and chest compressions
- Positive-pressure ventilation, chest compressions, and epinephrine

Endotracheal intubation also likely would have been performed. You would have checked the efficacy of each of the steps, and you would have considered the possibility of hypovolemia.

If the heart rate is detectable but remains below 60 bpm, it is still likely that the baby will respond to resuscitation, unless the baby is either extremely immature or has a lethal congenital malformation. If you are certain that effective ventilation, chest compressions, and medications are being provided, you might then consider mechanical causes of poor response, such as an airway malformation, pneumothorax, diaphragmatic hernia, or congenital heart disease (discussed in Lesson 7).

If the heart rate is absent, or no progress is being made in certain conditions, such as extreme prematurity, it may be appropriate to discontinue resuscitative efforts. You should be confident that optimum technique has been administered for a minimum of 10 minutes before considering such a decision. How long to continue and the ethical considerations involved will be discussed in Lesson 9.

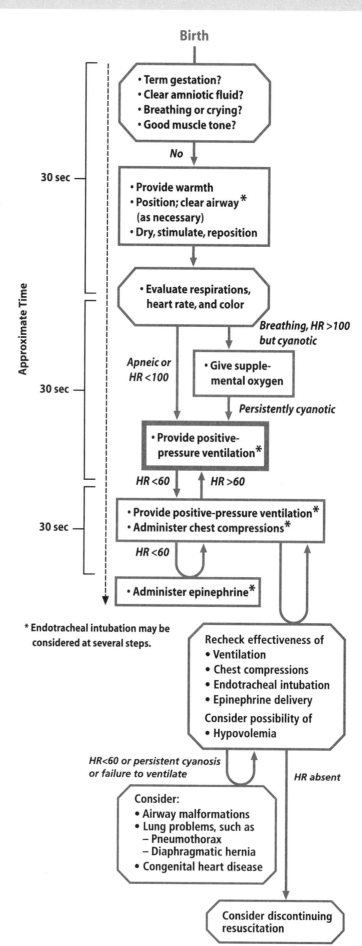

Key Points

1. Epinephrine, a cardiac stimulant, is indicated when the heart rate remains below 60 beats per minute, despite 30 seconds of assisted ventilation followed by another 30 seconds of coordinated chest compressions and ventilations.

2. Recommended epinephrine
   • Concentration: 1:10,000 (0.1 mg/mL)
   • Route: Intravenously. Endotracheal administration may be considered while intravenous access is being established.
   • Dose: 0.1 to 0.3 mL/kg (consider higher dose, 0.3 to 1 mL/kg, for endotracheal route only)
   • Preparation: 1:10,000 solution
   • Rate: *Rapidly*—as quickly as possible

3. Epinephrine should be given by umbilical vein. The endotracheal route is often faster and more accessible than placing an umbilical catheter, but is associated with unreliable absorption and may not be effective at the lower dose.

4. Indications for volume expansion during resuscitation include
   • Baby is not responding to resuscitation
   AND
   • Baby appears in shock (pale color, weak pulses, persistently low heart rate, no improvement in circulatory status despite resuscitation efforts)
   AND
   • There is a history of condition associated with fetal blood loss (eg, extensive vaginal bleeding, abruptio placentae, placenta previa, twin-to-twin transfusion, etc).

5. Recommended volume expander
   • Solution: Normal saline, Ringer's lactate, or O Rh-negative blood
   • Dose: 10 mL/kg
   • Route: Umbilical vein
   • Preparation: Correct volume drawn into large syringe
   • Rate: Over 5 to 10 minutes

Lesson 6 Review

(The answers follow.)

1. Fewer than _____ babies per 1,000 births will need epinephrine to stimulate their hearts.

2. As soon as you suspect that medications may be needed during a resuscitation, one member of the team should begin to insert an _____ to deliver the drug(s).

3. Effective ventilation and coordinated chest compressions have been performed for 30 seconds and the baby's heart rate is less than 60 beats per minute. You should now give _____ while continuing chest compressions and _____.

4. What is the problem with administering epinephrine through an endotracheal tube? _____

5. You should follow an intravenous dose of epinephrine with a flush of _____ to ensure that most of the drug is delivered to the baby and not left in the catheter.

6. Epinephrine (increases) (decreases) the strength of cardiac contractions and (increases) (decreases) the rate of cardiac contractions.

7. The recommended concentration of epinephrine for newborns is (1:1,000) (1:10,000).

8. The recommended dose of epinephrine for newborns is ___ to ___ mL/kg, if given intravenously, and ___ to ___ mL/kg, if given endotracheally, of a 1:10,000 solution.

9. Epinephrine should be given (slowly) (as quickly as possible).

10. What should you do approximately 30 seconds after giving epinephrine? _____

11. If the baby's heart rate remains below 60 beats per minute, you can repeat the dose of epinephrine every _____ to _____ minutes.

12. If the baby's heart rate remains below 60 beats per minute after you have given epinephrine, you also should check to make sure that ventilation is producing adequate lung inflation, and that _____ are being done correctly.

13. If the baby appears to be in shock, there is evidence of blood loss, and resuscitation is not resulting in improvement, you should consider giving _____ mL/kg of _____ by _____.

Answers to Questions

1. Fewer than **2** babies per 1,000 births will need epinephrine to stimulate their hearts.

2. One member of the team should begin to insert an **umbilical venous catheter** when you anticipate that drugs will be needed.

3. You should give **epinephrine** while continuing chest compressions and **ventilation.**

4. **Epinephrine is not reliably absorbed when given by the endotracheal route. A higher dose (0.3 to 1 mL/kg) should be considered if epinephrine is given while umbilical venous access is being established.**

5. You should follow an injection of epinephrine with a flush of **normal saline.**

6. Epinephrine **increases** the strength of cardiac contractions and **increases** the rate of cardiac contractions.

7. The recommended concentration of epinephrine for newborns is **1:10,000.**

8. The recommended dose of epinephrine for newborns is **0.1 to 0.3** mL/kg, if given intravenously, of a 1:10,000 solution. The recommended dose of epinephrine, if given endotracheally, is **0.3 to 1** mL/kg of a 1:10,000 solution.

9. Epinephrine should be given **as quickly as possible.**

10. You should **check the heart rate** approximately 30 seconds after giving epinephrine.

11. If the baby's heart rate remains below 60 beats per minute, you can repeat the dose of epinephrine every **3** to **5** minutes.

12. Check to make sure that ventilation is producing adequate lung inflation, and that **chest compressions** are being done correctly.

13. Consider giving **10** mL/kg of **volume expander** by **umbilical vein.**

Performance Checklist

Lesson 6 — Medications

Instructor: The learner should be instructed to talk through the procedure as it is demonstrated. Judge the performance of each step and check (✓) the box when the action is completed correctly. If done incorrectly, circle the box so that you can discuss that step later. You will need to provide information at several points concerning the condition of the baby.

Learner: To successfully complete this checklist, you should be able to perform all the steps and make all the correct decisions in the procedure. You should talk through the procedure as you perform it.

Equipment and Supplies

For epinephrine or volume expander via umbilical venous catheter:

Umbilical cord segment for cannulation (simulated or real)*

3-mL syringes

20-mL syringes

3-way stopcock

3.5F or 5F umbilical catheters

Normal saline flush

Antiseptic solution (or simulated)

Gloves

Umbilical tape

Scalpel handle and blade

Curved hemostat

Forceps

Epinephrine 1:10,000 (or simulation)

Normal saline for volume expansion (or simulation)

Needle

Medication labels

Code sheet for recording medication

* If using human umbilical cord segments:

Human umbilical cord stabilized in bottle nipple (see Instructor's Manual)

Personal protection equipment (barrier gown, gloves, face protection)

Appropriate disposal supplies (laundry bag, sharps container, biohazard bag)

For epinephrine via endotracheal tube:

Intubation manikin

Epinephrine 1:10,000 (or simulation)

3-mL or 5-mL syringes

Medication labels

Self-inflating bag with reservoir

or

Flow-inflating bag with oxygen source

Code sheet for recording medication

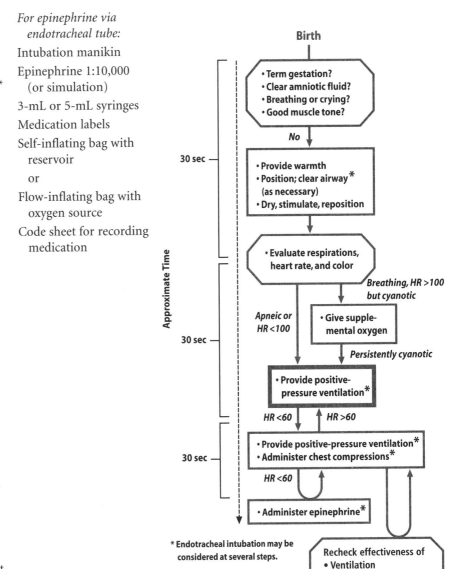

Performance Checklist

Lesson 6 — Medications via the umbilical vein

Name _____ Instructor _____ Date _____

The first part of this Performance Checklist is divided into 2 roles—inserting the catheter and preparing/administering medications. If only one learner is being evaluated, the learner may perform both roles or the instructor may take the role of the other person.

Instructor's statements are in quotes. Learner's questions and correct responses are in bold type. Instructor should check boxes as the learner answers correctly.

"A full-term newborn presented with poor muscle tone, apnea, and central cyanosis. She was placed under a radiant warmer. Resuscitation so far has included bag-and-mask ventilation, endotracheal intubation, and 30 seconds of chest compressions. The heart rate is still 30 bpm. Please demonstrate what you would do."

Inserts   Prepares

Prepares umbilical catheter for insertion

      Fills a 3-mL syringe with normal saline ☐

      Attaches 3-way stopcock to umbilical catheter ☐

      Flushes umbilical catheter and stopcock with normal saline ☐

      Closes the stopcock to the catheter to prevent loss of fluid and air entry into catheter ☐

☐ **Preps the base and lower few centimeters of the cord with appropriate antiseptic solution**

☐ **Ties umbilical tape loosely around base of cord**

☐ **Using sterile technique, cuts cord with scalpel to expose vein**

Positions umbilical venous catheter in umbilical vein

    ☐ **Inserts catheter into vein**

    Opens stopcock between baby and syringe and gently aspirates syringe to detect blood return ☐

    ☐ **Advances catheter until blood return is detected**

    Clears any air from catheter and stopcock ☐

☐ Asks for an estimate of baby's weight

"The baby appears to weigh about 3 kg."

☐ States that epinephrine is required and correct dose (0.1 to 0.3 mL/kg)

☐ Checks medication label for name of medication and concentration (Epinephrine: 1:10,000)

☐ Uses proper-sized syringe (1 mL)

☐ Calculates correct volume of epinephrine to be administered to this infant (0.3 to 0.9 mL)

☐ Draws up correct dose of epinephrine into 1-mL syringe and labels appropriately

☐ Prepares normal saline flush

☐ Double checks medication and dose by verbalizing medication and dose to be administered ☐

☐ Holds catheter in place as epinephrine is administered rapidly and with no accompanying air bubbles ☐

Flushes tubing to ensure proper dose ☐

☐ Listens to chest and reports heart rate

Records epinephrine dose, route, time, and newborn response on code sheet ☐

"This baby has responded well to your actions and now has a heart rate of 120 bpm and continues to improve. However, assume that the history had included profuse maternal vaginal bleeding and the heart rate remains 50 bpm, despite all that you have done so far. Describe what else you might consider and what additional actions might be required."

☐ Checks adequacy of positive-pressure ventilation and chest compressions and asks if the baby appears to be in shock (pale and with poor perfusion)

☐ States that she or he would consider giving a volume expander

"What would you use for a volume expander and how would you give it?"

☐ Describes using normal saline, Ringer's lactate, or O Rh-negative blood, if available

☐ Gives dose of 10 mL/kg

☐ Describes rate of infusion through umbilical catheter as over 5 to 10 minutes

"You now detect 12 beats in 6 seconds. Baby is still apneic."

Inserts   ## Prepares

☐ Indicates that chest compressions can stop, positive-pressure ventilation should continue, and catheter can be removed

☐ Removes catheter, secures umbilical tape, and monitors for bleeding at site

Overall

Understands technique to withdraw single dose of drug from original packaging ☐

Understands directional use of stopcock ☐

☐ Recognizes appropriate volume for drug or volume expander

Administers drug or volume expander over appropriate periods of time ☐

☐ Uses standard precautions and sterile technique

Performance Checklist

Lesson 6 — Epinephrine via the endotracheal tube

Name _____ Instructor _____ Date _____

This additional performance checklist addresses giving epinephrine down the endotracheal tube. As described in the lesson, endotracheal epinephrine has been shown to result in unpredictable blood levels and to produce an unreliable response in the baby. Nevertheless, in the real world, the immediate availability of sufficient personnel and the time required to establish an intravenous line have led some clinicians to want to give an endotracheal dose of epinephrine while the line is being established. This performance checklist is included to describe the technique of endotracheal administration and to emphasize the important differences in dosing for the endotracheal versus the intravenous route.

"A full-term newborn presented with poor muscle tone, apnea, and central cyanosis. She was placed under a radiant warmer. Resuscitation so far has included bag-and-mask ventilation, endotracheal intubation, and 30 seconds of chest compressions. The heart rate is still 30 bpm. While an umbilical line is being prepared, the decision is made to give an endotracheal dose of epinephrine. Please demonstrate what you would do."

☐ **Asks for an estimate of baby's weight**

"The baby appears to weigh about 3 kg."

☐ **States that epinephrine is required and correct dose**

☐ **Checks medication label for name of medication and concentration**

☐ **Uses proper-sized syringe (3 or 5 mL)**

☐ **Calculates correct volume of epinephrine to be administered to this infant (0.9 to 3 mL)**

☐ **Draws up correct dose of epinephrine into 3- or 5-mL syringe and labels appropriately**

☐ **Double checks medication and dose by verbalizing medication and dose to be administered**

☐ **Gives drug directly into the tube**
• Does not deposit medication into the connector

☐ **Provides ventilation after the drug is instilled**

☐ **Records medication, dose, route, time, and newborn response on code sheet**

Special Considerations

In Lesson 7 you will learn about

- Special situations that may complicate resuscitation and cause ongoing problems

- Subsequent management of the baby who has required resuscitation

- How the principles in this program can be applied to babies who require resuscitation beyond the immediate newborn period or outside the hospital delivery room

What complications should you consider if the baby still is not doing well after initial attempts at resuscitation?

You have learned that nearly all compromised newborns will respond to appropriate stimulation and measures to improve ventilation. A few may require chest compressions and medications to improve, and a very small number will die, despite all appropriate resuscitation measures.

However, another small group of newborns will respond initially to resuscitation but then remain compromised. These babies may have a congenital malformation or infection, or they may have experienced a complication of birth or of resuscitation. Sometimes you will know of the problem before birth as a result of antepartum ultrasound or some other method of antenatal diagnosis.

The continuing difficulty you encounter will be different for every baby, depending on the underlying problem. You may be unable to ventilate some babies, despite your best efforts to provide positive-pressure ventilation. Others may be easily ventilated but remain cyanotic or have a persistent low heart rate. Still other babies may fail to begin spontaneous breathing after you have given effective positive-pressure ventilation.

The most effective approach for babies who do not continue to improve after resuscitation will depend on their specific clinical presentation.

- Does positive-pressure ventilation fail to result in adequate ventilation of the lungs?

- Does the baby remain cyanotic or bradycardic, despite good ventilation?

- Does the baby fail to begin spontaneous respirations?

Each of these 3 questions will be addressed separately.

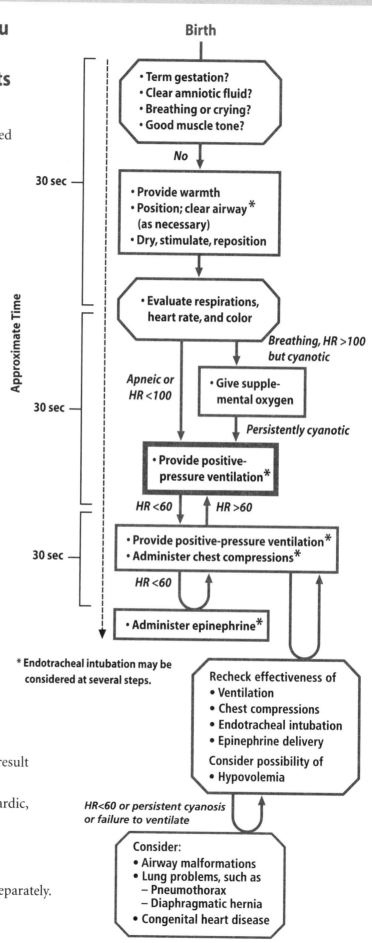

What if positive-pressure ventilation fails to result in adequate ventilation of the lungs?

If you have cleared the airway, positioned the baby's head correctly in the "sniffing" position, ensured a tight seal between the mask and the baby's face, and used sufficient positive-pressure ventilation, the heart rate, color, and tone should be improving. If there is still bradycardia, you should assure yourself that there is perceptible chest movement with each positive-pressure breath and, when you listen to the lungs with a stethoscope, you should hear good airflow in and out of the baby's lungs. If you fail to see chest movement and do not hear good airflow, one of the following may be the problem:

Mechanical blockage of the airway, perhaps from

- Meconium or mucus in the pharynx or trachea
- Choanal atresia
- Pharyngeal airway malformation (such as Robin syndrome)
- Other rare conditions (such as laryngeal web)

Impaired lung function, perhaps from

- Pneumothorax
- Congenital pleural effusions
- Congenital diaphragmatic hernia
- Pulmonary hypoplasia
- Extreme immaturity
- Congenital pneumonia

Mechanical blockage of the airway

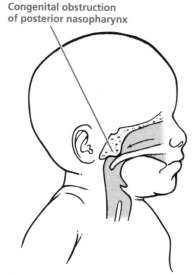

Congenital obstruction of posterior nasopharynx

Figure 7.1. Choanal atresia

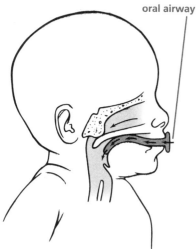

oral airway

Figure 7.2. Oral airway for choanal atresia

Meconium or mucus blockage

Remember that the airway has not been tested until the time of birth. If initial suctioning of meconium or simple noninvasive measures, such as head positioning and suctioning the mouth and nose, fail to establish an adequate airway, consider suctioning the airway deeper in the mouth and nose with a large suction catheter (size 10F or 12F).

The best way to rule out mucus or meconium in the airway is to insert an endotracheal tube and apply suction (as described in Lessons 2 and 5). Sometimes large plugs of meconium block the airway of a meconium-stained baby.

Choanal atresia

The anatomy of a baby's airway requires the nasal airway to be patent for air to reach the lungs during spontaneous breathing. Babies cannot breathe easily through their mouths unless they are actively crying. Therefore, if the nasal airway is filled with mucus or meconium, or if the nasal airway did not form properly (choanal atresia), the baby will have severe respiratory distress (Figure 7.1). Although choanal atresia generally will not prevent you from ventilating the baby with positive pressure through the oropharynx, the baby may not be able to move air spontaneously through the blocked nasopharynx.

Test for choanal atresia by passing a small-caliber suction catheter into the posterior pharynx through one, and then the other, naris. Direct the catheter perpendicular to the baby's face so that it will travel along the floor of the nasal passageway. If the catheter will not pass when directed correctly, choanal atresia may be present. You will need to insert a plastic oral airway to allow air to pass through the mouth (Figure 7.2), or you may use an endotracheal tube as the oral airway, passing it through the mouth and into the posterior pharynx, without having to insert it all the way into the trachea.

Pharyngeal airway malformation (Robin syndrome)

Some babies are born with a very small mandible, which results in a critical narrowing of the pharyngeal airway (Figure 7.3). During the first few months following birth, the mandible usually will grow to produce an adequate airway, but the baby may have considerable difficulty breathing immediately after birth. The main problem at birth is that the posteriorly placed tongue falls far back into the pharynx and obstructs the airway just above the larynx.

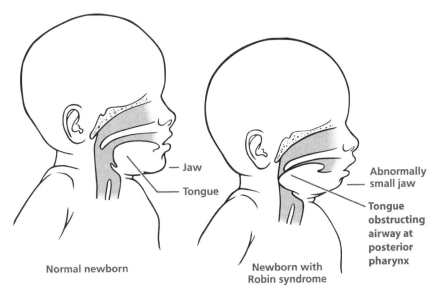

Figure 7.3. Normal newborn and newborn with Robin syndrome

Your first action should be to turn the baby onto his stomach (prone). This often allows the tongue to fall forward, thus opening the airway. If this is not successful, the next most effective means of achieving an airway for a baby with Robin syndrome is to insert a large catheter (12F) or small endotracheal tube (2.5 mm) through the nose, with the tip located deep in the posterior pharynx (Figure 7.4). This tube may relieve the suction that often causes the tongue to obstruct the airway. These 2 procedures (turning the baby prone and inserting a nasopharyngeal tube) usually permit the baby to move air well on his own without the need for positive-pressure ventilation.

 It is usually very difficult to place an endotracheal tube into the trachea of a baby with Robin syndrome. Prone positioning and a nasopharyngeal tube are often sufficient to maintain the airway.

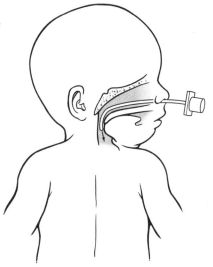

Figure 7.4. Prone positioning and placing a tube in posterior pharynx usually open the airway of a baby with Robin syndrome

If none of these procedures results in adequate air movement, and attempts at endotracheal intubation are unsuccessful, some clinicians have found placement of a laryngeal mask airway to be effective. (See Lesson 5.)

Other rare conditions
Congenital malformations, such as laryngeal webs, cystic hygroma, or congenital goiter, have been reported as rare causes of airway compromise in the newborn. Most, but not all, of these malformations will be evident by external examination of the baby. If an endotracheal tube cannot be passed, an emergency tracheostomy may be required. This procedure will not be described here.

Impaired lung function

Any substance that collects between the outside of the lung and the inside surface of the chest wall may prevent the lung from expanding within the chest. This causes respiratory distress and the baby may be persistently cyanotic and bradycardic.

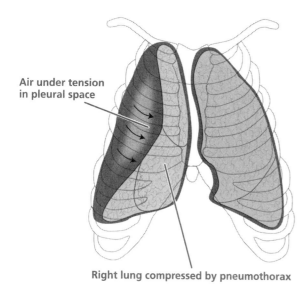

Air under tension in pleural space

Right lung compressed by pneumothorax

Figure 7.5. Pneumothorax compromising lung function

Pneumothorax

It is not uncommon for small air leaks to develop as the lung of the newborn fills with air. The likelihood is increased significantly if positive-pressure ventilation is required, particularly in the presence of meconium or a lung malformation, such as congenital diaphragmatic hernia. (See page 7-8.) Air that leaks from inside the lung and collects in the pleural space is called a pneumothorax (Figure 7.5). If the pneumothorax becomes large enough, the trapped air under tension can prevent the lung from expanding and also can block blood flow to the lung, resulting in respiratory distress, cyanosis, and bradycardia.

Breath sounds will be diminished on the side of the pneumothorax. Definitive diagnosis can be made with an x-ray. Transillumination of the chest may be helpful as a screening procedure.

 Caution: Loss of breath sounds on the left also may be a reflection of the endotracheal tube being in too far, down the right main stem bronchus.

If a pneumothorax causes significant respiratory distress, it should be relieved by placing a percutaneous catheter, needle, or chest tube into the pleural space (see page 7-7). A small pneumothorax will usually absorb spontaneously and may not require treatment.

Pleural effusions

Collections of fluid within the pleural space cause the same symptoms as a pneumothorax. In rare circumstances, edema fluid, chyle (lymph fluid), or blood collects in the pleural space of a newborn and prevents the lungs from adequately expanding. Usually other signs of problems, such as total-body edema (hydrops fetalis), are present in such newborns.

Diagnosis of fluid in the pleural space can be made by x-ray. If respiratory distress is significant, insert a percutaneous catheter, needle, or chest tube into the pleural space to drain the fluid, as described in the following text.

The details of how to place a chest tube surgically are beyond the scope of this program. However, in an emergency situation where the baby is in respiratory failure from a pneumothorax or pleural effusion, the air or fluid may be drained by percutaneous catheter or needle aspiration.

> **!** If a baby has worsening bradycardia and cyanosis and has asymmetric breath sounds after initial resuscitation, you may decide to emergently insert a percutaneous catheter or needle into the chest on the side of the decreased breath sounds while waiting for results of a chest x-ray.

The baby first should be turned on her side, with the pneumothorax side superior, to allow the air to rise. An 18-gauge or 20-gauge percutaneous catheter is inserted perpendicular to the chest wall and just over the top of the rib in the fourth intercostal space at the anterior axillary line on the suspected side (Figure 7.6 - top). The fourth intercostal space is located at the level of the nipples. The needle is then retracted and removed from the catheter, and a 3-way stopcock connected to a 20-mL syringe is connected to the catheter (Figure 7.6). The stopcock is then opened between the syringe and the catheter and the syringe is aspirated to remove air or fluid. When the syringe is full, the stopcock may be closed to the chest while the syringe is emptied. The stopcock then may be reopened to the chest and more fluid or air aspirated until the baby's condition has improved. An x-ray should be obtained to document the presence or absence of residual pneumothorax or effusion.

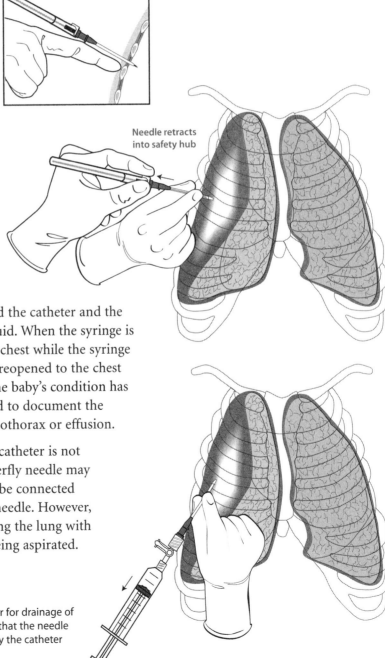

Needle retracts into safety hub

If an appropriate-gauge percutaneous catheter is not available, a 19-gauge or 21-gauge butterfly needle may be used. In this case, the stopcock can be connected directly to the tubing of the butterfly needle. However, there is a small possibility of puncturing the lung with the butterfly needle as fluid or air is being aspirated.

Figure 7.6. Insertion of a percutaneous catheter for drainage of a pneumothorax or pleural fluid (see text). Note that the needle has been removed in the lower drawing and only the catheter remains in the pleural space

Congenital diaphragmatic hernia

The diaphragm normally separates the abdominal contents from the thoracic contents. When the diaphragm does not form completely, some of the abdominal contents (usually the intestines and the stomach, and sometimes the liver) enter the chest and prevent the lung on that side from developing normally. A diaphragmatic hernia often can be diagnosed by ultrasound before birth. Without antenatal diagnosis, the baby with a diaphragmatic hernia may present at birth with completely unanticipated respiratory distress.

A baby with a diaphragmatic hernia often presents with persistent respiratory distress and often has an unusually flat-appearing (scaphoid) abdomen, because the abdomen has less contents than normal. Breath sounds are diminished on the side of the hernia. These babies also have persistent pulmonary hypertension and, therefore, may remain persistently cyanotic from poor pulmonary blood flow.

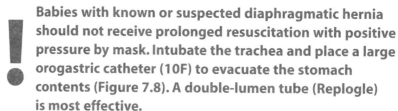

Figure 7.7. Compromised lung function from presence of a congenital diaphragmatic hernia

When the baby is born, the underdeveloped lung cannot expand normally. If positive pressure is delivered by mask during resuscitation, some of the positive-pressure gas enters the stomach and intestines (Figure 7.7). Because the intestines are in the chest, lung inflation is increasingly inhibited. Also, positive pressure delivered to the underdeveloped lung may result in a pneumothorax.

> **!** Babies with known or suspected diaphragmatic hernia should not receive prolonged resuscitation with positive pressure by mask. Intubate the trachea and place a large orogastric catheter (10F) to evacuate the stomach contents (Figure 7.8). A double-lumen tube (Replogle) is most effective.

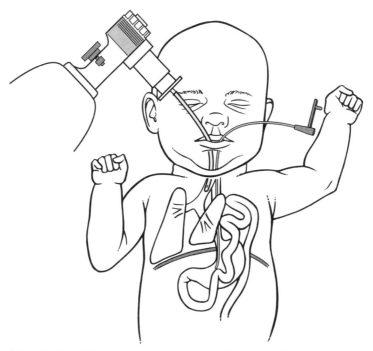

Figure 7.8. Stabilizing treatment for baby with diaphragmatic hernia (endotracheal tube in place and tube in stomach)

Pulmonary hypoplasia

Normal lung development requires the presence of amniotic fluid. Any condition that causes severe oligohydramnios (such as renal agenesis) may result in pulmonary hypoplasia. High inflation pressures will be required and pneumothoraces are common. Severe pulmonary hypoplasia usually is incompatible with survival.

Extreme immaturity

Babies with extremely immature lungs may be very difficult to ventilate, even with very high inflation pressures. (See Lesson 8.)

Congenital pneumonia

Although congenital pneumonia usually presents as worsening lung disease after birth, some overwhelming infections (such as group B streptococcal disease) may present as respiratory failure at birth. Also, aspiration of amniotic fluid, particularly if contaminated with meconium, can cause severe respiratory compromise.

What if the baby remains cyanotic or bradycardic despite good ventilation?

First, ensure that the baby's chest is moving adequately, that you can hear good equal breath sounds on both sides of the chest, and that 100% oxygen is being given. If the baby still is bradycardic and/or cyanotic, he may have congenital heart disease. Confirmation with a chest x-ray, an electrocardiogram, and/or an echocardiogram may be necessary. However, remember that congenital heart block or even cyanotic congenital heart disease are rare conditions, while inadequate ventilation following birth is a much more common cause of persistent cyanosis and bradycardia.

 Babies with congenital heart disease are seldom critically ill immediately following birth. Problems with resuscitation are almost always due to failure to successfully ventilate.

What if the baby fails to begin spontaneous respirations?

If positive-pressure ventilation has resulted in heart rate and color improving to normal but the baby still has poor muscle tone and fails to breathe spontaneously, the baby may have depressed brain or muscle activity due to

- Brain injury (hypoxic-ischemic encephalopathy [HIE]), severe acidosis, or a congenital neuromuscular disorder

or

- Sedation due to drugs previously administered to the mother and passed to the baby across the placenta

Narcotics given to the laboring mother to relieve pain also may inhibit respiratory drive and activity in the newborn. In such cases, administration of naloxone (a narcotic antagonist) to the newborn will reverse the effect of narcotics on the baby.

 Giving a narcotic antagonist is not the correct first therapy for a baby who is not breathing. The first corrective action is positive-pressure ventilation.

Naloxone Hydrochloride

Recommended concentration =
1.0-mg/mL solution

Recommended route =
Intravenous preferred; intramuscular acceptable, but delayed onset of action. There are no studies reporting the efficacy of endotracheal naloxone.

Recommended dose =
0.1 mg/kg

*The indications for giving **naloxone** to the baby require both of the following to be present:*

- Continued respiratory depression after positive-pressure ventilation has restored a normal heart rate and color

and

- A history of maternal narcotic administration within the past 4 hours

After naloxone administration, continue to administer positive-pressure ventilation until the baby is breathing normally. The duration of action of the narcotic often exceeds that of naloxone, necessitating repeated doses of naloxone. Therefore, observe the baby closely for recurrent respiratory depression, necessitating repeated doses of naloxone.

 Caution: Do not give naloxone to the newborn of a mother who is suspected of being addicted to narcotics or is on methadone maintenance. This may result in the newborn having seizures.

Other drugs given to the mother, such as magnesium sulfate or non-narcotic analgesics or general anesthetics, also can depress respirations in the newborn and will not respond to naloxone. If maternal narcotics were not given to the mother or if naloxone does not result in restoring spontaneous respirations, transport the baby to the nursery for further evaluation and management while continuing to administer positive-pressure ventilation.

Review

(The answers are in the preceding section and at the end of the lesson.)

1. Choanal atresia can be ruled out by what procedure?

   _____

2. Babies with Robin syndrome who have upper airway obstruction
   may be helped by placing a _____
   and positioning them _____.
   Endotracheal intubation of such babies is usually (easy) (difficult).

3. A pneumothorax or congenital diaphragmatic hernia should be
   considered if breath sounds are (equal) (unequal) on different
   sides of the chest.

4. You should suspect a congenital diaphragmatic hernia if the
   abdomen is _____. Such babies
   should not be resuscitated with _____.

5. Persistent bradycardia and cyanosis during resuscitation most likely
   are caused by (heart problems) (inadequate ventilation).

6. Babies who do not have spontaneous respirations and whose
   mothers have been given narcotic drugs should first receive
   _____ and then, if
   spontaneous respirations do not begin, may be given
   _____.

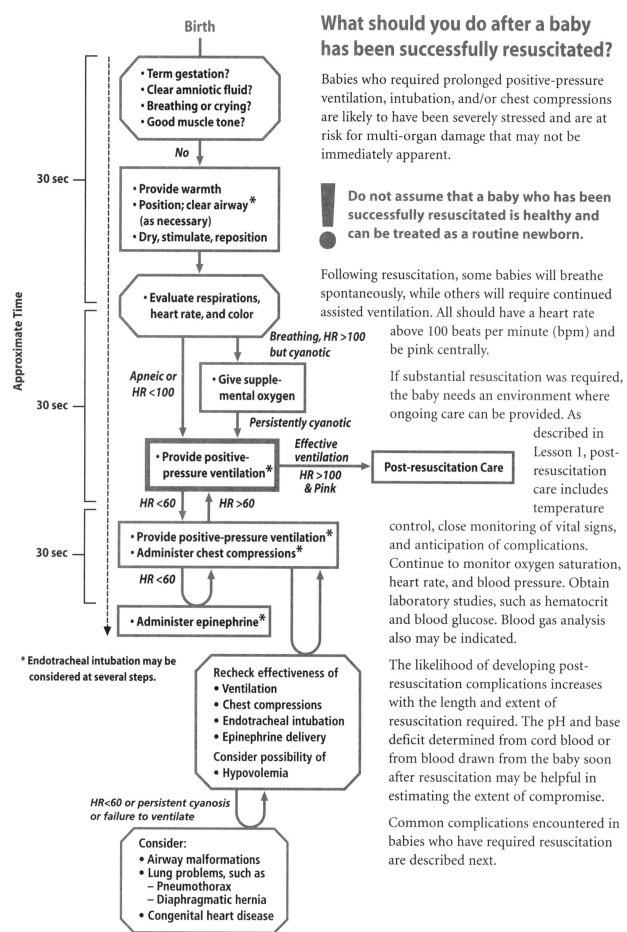

Birth

- Term gestation?
- Clear amniotic fluid?
- Breathing or crying?
- Good muscle tone?

No

30 sec

- Provide warmth
- Position; clear airway*
  (as necessary)
- Dry, stimulate, reposition

- Evaluate respirations,
  heart rate, and color

*Breathing, HR >100
but cyanotic*

*Apneic or
HR <100*

- Give supple-
  mental oxygen

30 sec

Persistently cyanotic

*Effective
ventilation*

- Provide positive-
  pressure ventilation*

*HR >100
& Pink*

Post-resuscitation Care

HR <60   *HR >60*

- Provide positive-pressure ventilation*
- Administer chest compressions*

30 sec

HR <60

- Administer epinephrine*

* Endotracheal intubation may be
considered at several steps.

Recheck effectiveness of
- Ventilation
- Chest compressions
- Endotracheal intubation
- Epinephrine delivery

Consider possibility of
- Hypovolemia

*HR<60 or persistent cyanosis
or failure to ventilate*

Consider:
- Airway malformations
- Lung problems, such as
  – Pneumothorax
  – Diaphragmatic hernia
- Congenital heart disease

Approximate Time

What should you do after a baby has been successfully resuscitated?

Babies who required prolonged positive-pressure ventilation, intubation, and/or chest compressions are likely to have been severely stressed and are at risk for multi-organ damage that may not be immediately apparent.

Do not assume that a baby who has been successfully resuscitated is healthy and can be treated as a routine newborn.

Following resuscitation, some babies will breathe spontaneously, while others will require continued assisted ventilation. All should have a heart rate above 100 beats per minute (bpm) and be pink centrally.

If substantial resuscitation was required, the baby needs an environment where ongoing care can be provided. As described in Lesson 1, post-resuscitation care includes temperature control, close monitoring of vital signs, and anticipation of complications. Continue to monitor oxygen saturation, heart rate, and blood pressure. Obtain laboratory studies, such as hematocrit and blood glucose. Blood gas analysis also may be indicated.

The likelihood of developing post-resuscitation complications increases with the length and extent of resuscitation required. The pH and base deficit determined from cord blood or from blood drawn from the baby soon after resuscitation may be helpful in estimating the extent of compromise.

Common complications encountered in babies who have required resuscitation are described next.

Pulmonary hypertension

As explained in Lesson 1, the blood vessels in the lungs are tightly constricted in the fetus. Ventilation and oxygenation at birth are the main stimuli that cause the blood vessels to relax, thus bringing blood to the lungs to pick up oxygen.

The pulmonary blood vessels in babies who have been extremely stressed at birth may remain constricted, thus resulting in hypoxemia due to pulmonary hypertension and requiring oxygen therapy. Severe pulmonary hypertension results in further hypoxemia and may require tertiary-level therapies, such as inhaled nitric oxide or extracorporeal membrane oxygenation (ECMO).

Additional pulmonary vasoconstriction may be prevented by avoiding episodes of hypoxemia after a baby has been resuscitated.

 Use an oximeter and/or arterial blood gas determinations to be certain that a baby who required resuscitation remains adequately oxygenated.

Pneumonia and other lung complications

Babies who require resuscitation are at higher risk for developing pneumonia, either from aspiration syndrome or from a congenital infection that may have been responsible for causing the perinatal compromise. Neonatal pneumonia also is associated with pulmonary hypertension.

If a baby who required resuscitation continues to show any ongoing signs of respiratory distress or requirement for supplemental oxygen, consider evaluating the baby for pneumonia or bacterial sepsis and beginning parenteral antibiotics.

If acute respiratory deterioration occurs during or after resuscitation, consider the possibility that the baby may have developed a pneumothorax; or, if the baby has remained intubated after resuscitation, consider the possibility of a dislodged or plugged endotracheal tube.

Metabolic acidosis

Although the use of sodium bicarbonate during resuscitation is controversial, it may be helpful to correct metabolic acidosis that results from a buildup of lactic acid. Lactic acid forms when tissues have insufficient oxygen. Severe acidosis causes the myocardium to contract poorly and causes the blood vessels of the lungs to constrict, thus decreasing pulmonary blood flow and preventing the lungs from adequately oxygenating the blood.

However, sodium bicarbonate can be harmful, particularly if given too early in a resuscitation. Be certain that ventilation of the lungs is adequate. When sodium bicarbonate mixes with acid, carbon dioxide (CO_2) is formed. The lungs must be adequately ventilated to remove the CO_2.

Do not give sodium bicarbonate unless the lungs are being adequately ventilated.

If you decide to give sodium bicarbonate, remember that it is very caustic and hypertonic and, therefore, must be given into a large vein, from which there is good blood return. The usual dose is 2 mEq/kg/dose, given as a 4.2% solution (0.5 mEq/mL) at a rate no faster than 1 mEq/kg/min.

 Sodium bicarbonate is very caustic and is NEVER given through the endotracheal tube during resuscitation.

Hypotension

Perinatal compromise can result in an insult to the heart muscle and/or to decreased vascular tone, resulting in hypotension. Heart murmurs often are audible from transient tricuspid insufficiency, which may reflect decreased right ventricular output. If sepsis or blood loss is the reason that the baby required resuscitation, the effective circulating blood volume may be low, which also can result in hypotension.

Babies who require resuscitation should have heart rate and blood pressure monitoring until blood pressure and peripheral perfusion are normal and stable. Blood transfusion or other volume expansion may be indicated, as described in Lesson 6, and some babies may require an infusion of an inotropic agent, such as dopamine, to assist cardiac output and vascular tone if the initial volume bolus does not result in normalization of blood pressure.

Fluid management

Perinatal compromise can result in renal dysfunction, which is usually transient (acute tubular necrosis) but can cause severe electrolyte and fluid shifts. Consider checking the urine for blood and protein to rule out acute tubular necrosis. Some severely depressed newborns also may develop a syndrome of inappropriate antidiuretic hormone secretion (SIADH). After severe perinatal compromise, urine output, body weight, and serum electrolyte levels should be checked frequently for the first few days after birth. Some may need their fluid and electrolyte intakes restricted until renal function returns to normal or SIADH resolves. Supplemental calcium may be required. Electrolyte abnormalities increase the risk of cardiac arrhythmias.

Seizures or apnea

Newborns who have perinatal compromise and undergo resuscitation may later manifest symptoms of HIE. Initially, the baby may have depressed muscle tone, but seizures may appear after several hours. Apnea or hypoventilation may also be a reflection of HIE.

These same symptoms also may be a manifestation of metabolic abnormalities (such as hypoglycemia) or electrolyte disturbances (such as hyponatremia or hypocalcemia).

Babies who have required extensive resuscitation should be monitored closely for seizures. Glucose and/or electrolyte therapy (per intravenous line) may be required. For seizures thought to be associated with HIE, anticonvulsant therapy (such as phenobarbital) may be required.

Hypoglycemia

Metabolism under conditions of oxygen deprivation, which may occur during perinatal compromise, consumes much more glucose than the same metabolism occurring in the presence of adequate oxygen. Although, initially, catecholamine secretion causes elevated serum glucose, glucose stores (glycogen) are depleted rapidly during perinatal compromise, and hypoglycemia may result. Glucose is an essential fuel for brain function in newborns.

Babies who require resuscitation need their blood glucose levels checked soon after resuscitation and then sequentially, until several values are within normal limits and adequate glucose intake is ensured. Intravenous glucose is often necessary to treat hypoglycemia.

Feeding problems

The gastrointestinal tract of a newborn is very sensitive to hypoxia-ischemia. Ileus, gastrointestinal bleeding, and even necrotizing enterocolitis can result. Also, because of neurologic insult, sucking patterns and coordination of sucking, swallowing, and breathing may take several days to recover. Intravenous fluids and nutrition may be required during this time.

Temperature management

Babies who have been resuscitated can become cold for a variety of reasons. Special techniques for maintaining normal body temperature in premature babies are addressed in Lesson 8. Other babies, in particular those born to mothers with chorioamnionitis, may have an elevated temperature in the delivery room. Since hyperthermia can be injurious to a baby, it is important not to overheat the baby during and following resuscitation. Babies' temperatures should be maintained in the normal range.

 Hyperthermia (overheating) can be very injurious to a baby. Be careful not to overheat the baby during or following resuscitation.

The statement above should not be confused with recent studies that have evaluated the potential neuroprotective role of modest hypothermia in near-term and term babies at high risk for progressing to HIE. Until this research is complete, maintaining a normal body temperature during and following resuscitation is advised.

Post-resuscitation Care

Organ System	Potential Complication	Post-resuscitation Action
Brain	Apnea Seizures	Monitor for apnea Support ventilation as needed Monitor glucose and electrolytes Avoid hyperthermia Consider anticonvulsant therapy
Lungs	Pulmonary hypertension Pneumonia Pneumothorax Transient tachypnea Meconium aspiration syndrome Surfactant deficiency	Maintain adequate oxygenation and ventilation Consider antibiotics Obtain x-ray if respiratory distress Consider surfactant therapy Delay feedings if respiratory distress
Cardiovascular	Hypotension	Monitor blood pressure and heart rate Consider inotrope (eg, dopamine) and/or volume replacement
Kidneys	Acute tubular necrosis	Monitor urine output Restrict fluids if baby is oliguric and vascular volume is adequate Monitor serum electrolytes
Gastrointestinal	Ileus Necrotizing enterocolitis	Delay initiation of feedings Give intravenous fluids Consider parenteral nutrition
Metabolic/ Hematologic	Hypoglycemia Hypocalcemia; hyponatremia Anemia Thrombocytopenia	Monitor blood glucose Monitor electrolytes Monitor hematocrit Monitor platelets

Review

(The answers are in the preceding section and at the end of the lesson.)

7. After resuscitation of a term or near-term newborn, blood pressure in the pulmonary circuit is more likely to be (high) (low). Adequate oxygenation is likely to cause the pulmonary blood flow to (increase) (decrease).

8. If a meconium-stained baby has been resuscitated and then develops acute deterioration, a _____ should be suspected.

9. A baby who required resuscitation still has low blood pressure and poor perfusion after having been given a blood transfusion for suspected perinatal blood loss. He may require an infusion of _____ to improve his cardiac output and vascular tone.

10. Babies who have been resuscitated may have suffered kidney damage and are more likely to need (more) (less) fluids after the resuscitation.

11. A baby has a seizure 10 hours after being resuscitated. A blood glucose screen and serum electrolytes are normal. What class of drug should be used to treat her seizure?

    _____

12. List 3 causes of seizures following resuscitation.
    (1) _____
    (2) _____
    (3) _____

13. Because energy stores are consumed faster in the absence of oxygen, blood _____ levels may be low following resuscitation.

Are the resuscitation techniques different for babies born outside the hospital or beyond the immediate newborn period?

Throughout this program, you have learned about resuscitating newly born babies who were born in the hospital and were having difficulty making the transition from intrauterine to extrauterine life. Some babies, of course, may encounter difficulty and require resuscitation after being born outside of the hospital, and other babies will require resuscitation beyond the immediate newborn period.

Some examples of babies who may require resuscitation under different circumstances include

- A baby who delivers precipitously at home or in a motor vehicle, where resources are limited.
- A baby who develops apnea in the nursery.
- A 2-day-old baby with sepsis who presents in shock.
- An intubated baby in the neonatal intensive care unit who deteriorates acutely. (Babies requiring resuscitation in this situation have a mechanical problem with the endotracheal tube or ventilator more often than a new onset medical problem. The resuscitation team should remove the baby from the ventilator and hand ventilate the baby's lungs while the problem is investigated and treated.)

Although scenarios outside the delivery room are different, the physiologic principles and the steps you take to restore vital signs during the newborn period (first month after birth) remain the same.

- Warm, position, clear airway, stimulate the baby to breathe, and give oxygen (as necessary).
- Establish effective ventilation.
- Provide chest compressions.
- Administer medications.

 The priority for resuscitating babies at any time during the newborn period, regardless of location, should be to restore adequate ventilation.

Once adequate ventilation is ensured, consider any available information about the baby's history to guide the focus of your resuscitation efforts.

Although this program is not designed to teach neonatal resuscitation in these other venues, some strategies for applying the principles outside the delivery room are presented in the next few pages. More details are available through other programs, such as the Pediatric Advanced Life Support (PALS) program of the American Heart Association or the Pediatric Education for Prehospital Professionals (PEPP) program of the American Academy of Pediatrics.

Case 7.
Resuscitation of an apparently healthy newborn

A baby weighing 3,400 g is born in the hospital at term after an uncomplicated pregnancy, labor, and delivery. The transitional period is uneventful; he remains with his mother and begins breastfeeding soon after birth.

At approximately 20 hours of age, his mother finds him apneic and unresponsive in his bassinet. She activates the emergency alarm, and a perinatal nurse on the floor responds immediately.

The nurse finds the baby apneic, limp, and blue. She places him under a radiant warmer, and opens his airway by placing his head in the "sniffing" position. She quickly suctions his mouth and nose with a bulb syringe. She rubs his back and flicks the soles of his feet but he still does not resume breathing. The nurse calls for help.

A self-inflating resuscitation bag and mask is readily available and used to deliver positive-pressure ventilation. A second nurse arrives to help and attaches the bag to 100% oxygen. After approximately 30 seconds of positive-pressure ventilation, the second nurse uses a stethoscope to check the heart rate and finds it to be 30 bpm.

Chest compressions are started and coordinated with positive-pressure ventilation. After 30 seconds, the heart rate is checked again and found to be 40 bpm. A third clinician arrives and inserts an endotracheal tube. An intravenous line is inserted and 1 mL of 1:10,000 epinephrine is administered into the line. After another 30 seconds, the heart rate is found to be 80 bpm.

Chest compressions are discontinued, and positive-pressure ventilation continues. After another minute, the heart rate increases to more than 100 bpm, and the baby begins breathing spontaneously.

A pulse oximeter is placed and the baby is moved to a transport incubator. A nurse provides support and information to the anxious mother as the baby is moved to the nursery for evaluation of the cause of his respiratory arrest.

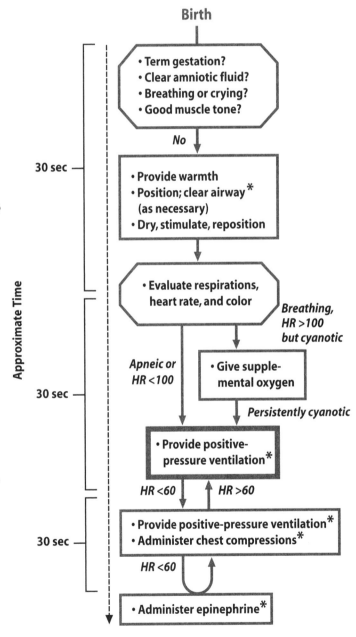

Birth

- Term gestation?
- Clear amniotic fluid?
- Breathing or crying?
- Good muscle tone?

No

30 sec

- Provide warmth
- Position; clear airway* (as necessary)
- Dry, stimulate, reposition

- Evaluate respirations, heart rate, and color

Breathing, HR >100 but cyanotic

Apneic or HR <100

- Give supplemental oxygen

Persistently cyanotic

30 sec

- Provide positive-pressure ventilation*

HR <60   *HR >60*

- Provide positive-pressure ventilation*
- Administer chest compressions*

30 sec

HR <60

- Administer epinephrine*

* Endotracheal intubation may be considered at several steps.

Approximate Time

7-19

What are some of the different strategies needed to resuscitate outside the hospital or beyond the immediate newborn period?

Temperature control

Maintaining normal body temperature during resuscitation remains an important concept, but it becomes less difficult if the baby is not newly born, because the baby's entire body generally will not be wet. If the baby is newly born and requires resuscitation outside of the hospital, maintaining body temperature may become a major challenge, because you likely will not have a radiant warmer readily available. Some suggestions for minimizing heat loss are as follows:

- Turn up the heat source in the room or vehicle.

- Dry the baby well with bath towels, a blanket, or clean clothing.

- Use the mother's body as a heat source. Consider placing the baby skin-to-skin on the mother's chest and covering both baby and mother with a blanket.

Clearing the airway

If resuscitation is required outside a delivery room or nursery, vacuum suction will often not be readily available. Suggestions for methods of clearing the airway are as follows:

- Use a bulb syringe.

- Wipe the mouth and nose with a clean handkerchief or other cloth wrapped around your index finger.

Ventilation

Most babies breathe spontaneously after birth. Drying the newborn, rubbing his back, and flicking the soles of the feet are acceptable methods of stimulation. However, some babies born outside the hospital may require positive-pressure ventilation to ventilate the lungs. If a resuscitation bag-and-mask device is unavailable, positive-pressure ventilation can be delivered by mouth-to-mouth-and-nose. The baby is placed in the "sniffing" position, and the resuscitator's mouth should make a tight seal over the baby's mouth and nose. With particularly large babies or small-mouthed resuscitators, it may be necessary to cover only the baby's mouth with the resuscitator's mouth while the baby's nose is pinched to seal the airway. This technique poses a risk of transmission of infectious diseases.

Vascular access

Catheterization of the umbilical vessels is generally not an option outside the hospital or beyond the first several days after birth. In such cases, prompt cannulation of a peripheral vein or insertion of an intraosseus needle into the tibia are reasonable alternatives. Detailed description of these techniques is beyond the scope of this program.

Medications

Epinephrine should still be the primary drug used for resuscitation of babies who do not respond to positive-pressure ventilation and chest compressions. However, other medications (such as calcium) also may be necessary, depending on the cause of the arrest. The diagnostic steps required and the details of using these drugs are beyond the scope of this program.

Review

(The answers are in the preceding section and at the end of the lesson.)

14. You are likely to have (more) (less) (about the same) difficulty controlling body temperature of babies requiring resuscitation beyond the immediate newborn period.

15. The priority for resuscitating babies beyond the immediate newborn period should be to
    A. Defibrillate the heart
    B. Expand blood volume
    C. Establish effective ventilation
    D. Administer epinephrine
    E. Deliver chest compressions

16. If vacuum suction is not available to clear the airway, 2 alternative methods are _____ and _____.

17. If a 15-day-old baby requiring resuscitation had blood loss, vascular access routes include _____ and _____.

Key Points

1. The appropriate action for a baby who fails to respond to resuscitation will depend on the presentation—failure to ventilate, persistent cyanosis or bradycardia, or failure to initiate spontaneous breathing.

2. Symptoms from choanal atresia can be helped by placing an oral airway.

3. Airway obstruction from Robin syndrome can be helped by inserting a nasopharyngeal tube and placing the baby prone.

4. In an emergency, a pneumothorax can be detected by transillumination and treated by inserting a needle in the chest.

5. If diaphragmatic hernia is suspected, avoid positive-pressure ventilation by mask. Immediately intubate the trachea and insert an orogastric tube.

6. Persistent cyanosis and bradycardia are rarely caused by congenital heart disease. More commonly, the persistent cyanosis and bradycardia are caused by inadequate ventilation.

7. A baby who has required resuscitation must have close monitoring and management of oxygenation, infection, blood pressure, fluids, apnea, blood sugar, feeding, and temperature.

8. Be careful not to overheat the baby during or following resuscitation.

9. If a mother has recently received narcotics and her baby fails to breathe, first assist ventilation with positive pressure, then consider giving naloxone to the baby.

10. Restoring adequate ventilation remains the priority when resuscitating babies at birth in the delivery room or later in the nursery or other location.

11. Some alternative techniques for resuscitation outside of the delivery room include the following:
    - Maintain temperature by placing the baby skin-to-skin with the mother and raising the environmental temperature.
    - Clear airway with a bulb syringe or cloth on your finger.
    - Consider mouth-to-mouth-and-nose for administering positive pressure.
    - Cannulation of a peripheral vein or intraosseous space can be used for vascular access.

Lesson 7 Review

(The answers follow.)

1. Choanal atresia can be ruled out by what procedure?

   _____

2. Babies with Robin syndrome who have upper airway obstruction
   may be helped by placing a _____
   and positioning them _____.
   Endotracheal intubation of such babies is usually (easy) (difficult).

3. A pneumothorax or congenital diaphragmatic hernia should be
   considered if breath sounds are (equal) (unequal) on different
   sides of the chest.

4. You should suspect a congenital diaphragmatic hernia if the
   abdomen is _____. Such babies should
   not be resuscitated with _____.

5. Persistent bradycardia and cyanosis during resuscitation most likely
   are caused by (heart problems) (inadequate ventilation).

6. Babies who do not have spontaneous respirations and whose
   mothers have been given narcotic drugs should first receive
   _____ and then, if
   spontaneous respirations do not begin, may be given
   _____.

7. After resuscitation of a term or near-term newborn, blood pressure
   in the pulmonary circuit is more likely to be (high) (low).
   Adequate oxygenation is likely to cause the pulmonary blood flow
   to (increase) (decrease).

8. If a meconium-stained baby has been resuscitated and then
   develops acute deterioration, a _____
   should be suspected.

9. A baby who required resuscitation still has low blood pressure and
   poor perfusion after having been given a blood transfusion for
   suspected perinatal blood loss. He may require an infusion of
   _____ to improve his cardiac output and
   vascular tone.

Lesson 7 Review — *continued*

10. Babies who have been resuscitated may have suffered kidney damage and are more likely to need (more) (less) fluids after the resuscitation.

11. A baby has a seizure 10 hours after being resuscitated. A blood glucose screen and serum electrolytes are normal. What class of drug should be used to treat her seizure?

    _____

12. List 3 causes of seizures following resuscitation.

    (1) _____

    (2) _____

    (3) _____

13. Because energy stores are consumed faster in the absence of oxygen, blood _____ levels may be low following resuscitation.

14. You are likely to have (more) (less) (about the same) difficulty controlling body temperature of babies requiring resuscitation beyond the immediate newborn period.

15. The priority for resuscitating babies beyond the immediate newborn period should be to
    A. Defibrillate the heart
    B. Expand blood volume
    C. Establish effective ventilation
    D. Administer epinephrine
    E. Deliver chest compressions

16. If vacuum suction is not available to clear the airway, 2 alternative methods are _____ and
    _____.

17. If a 15-day-old baby requiring resuscitation had blood loss, vascular access routes include _____
    and _____.

Answers to Questions

1. Choanal atresia can be ruled out by **passing a nasopharyngeal catheter through the nares.**

2. Babies with Robin syndrome who have upper airway obstruction may be helped by placing a **nasopharyngeal tube** and positioning them **on their abdomens (prone).** Endotracheal intubation of such babies is usually **difficult.**

3. A pneumothorax or congenital diaphragmatic hernia should be considered if breath sounds are **unequal** on different sides of the chest. If the trachea has been intubated, you also should check to be sure that the tube is not in too far.

4. You should suspect a congenital diaphragmatic hernia if the abdomen is **flat-appearing (scaphoid).** Such babies should not be resuscitated with **positive-pressure ventilation by mask.**

5. Persistent bradycardia and cyanosis during resuscitation most likely are caused by **inadequate ventilation.**

6. Babies who do not have spontaneous respirations and whose mothers have been given narcotic drugs should first receive **positive-pressure ventilation** and then, if spontaneous respirations do not begin, may be given **naloxone.**

7. After resuscitation of a term or near-term newborn, blood pressure in the pulmonary circuit is more likely to be **high.** Adequate oxygenation is likely to cause the pulmonary vascular resistance to fall, and thus blood flow to **increase.**

8. If a meconium-stained baby has been resuscitated and then develops acute deterioration, a **pneumothorax** should be suspected. (An endotracheal tube plugged with meconium is also a consideration.)

9. The baby may require an infusion of **dopamine (or other inotrope)** to improve his cardiac output and vascular tone.

10. Babies who have been resuscitated are more likely to need **less** fluids after the resuscitation.

11. A baby with a seizure 10 hours after being resuscitated and with a normal blood sugar should be treated with **an anticonvulsant (such as phenobarbital).**

12. Seizures following resuscitation may be caused by (1) **hypoxic-ischemic encephalopathy,** (2) **metabolic disturbance, such as hypoglycemia,** or (3) **electrolyte abnormalities, such as hyponatremia or hypocalcemia.**

13. Blood **sugar (glucose)** levels may be low following resuscitation.

14. You are likely to have **less** difficulty controlling body temperature of babies requiring resuscitation beyond the immediate newborn period, since they usually will not be wet.

15. The priority for resuscitating babies beyond the immediate newborn period should be to **establish effective ventilation.**

16. If vacuum suction is not available to clear the airway, 2 alternative methods are **bulb suction** and **wiping the airway with a clean cloth.**

17. If a 15-day-old baby requiring resuscitation had blood loss, vascular access routes include **cannulation of a peripheral vein** and **insertion of an intraosseus needle.**

Resuscitation of Babies Born Preterm

In Lesson 8 you will learn

- The risk factors associated with being born preterm
- The additional resources needed to be prepared for a preterm delivery
- Additional strategies to maintain the preterm baby's body temperature
- Additional considerations for managing oxygen in a premature baby
- How to assist ventilation when a premature baby has difficulty breathing
- Ways to decrease the chances of brain injury
- Special precautions to take after resuscitating a premature baby

The following case describes the delivery and resuscitation of an extremely preterm baby. As you read the case, imagine yourself as part of the team from the anticipation of the delivery, through the resuscitation and stabilization and final transfer to an intensive care nursery.

Case 8.
Resuscitation and stabilization of a baby born extremely preterm

A 24-year-old woman is admitted to the obstetrical floor in early labor at 26 weeks' gestation. The expectant mother reports that contractions began approximately 6 hours ago. She also reports that membranes ruptured just before her arrival and that the fluid was bloody.

On admission, her cervix is 6-cm dilated, a fetal foot is palpable, and delivery is judged to be imminent. Because of breech presentation, a decision is made to deliver by cesarean section. A team with experience in neonatal resuscitation, including individuals with intubation and umbilical catheterization skills, is called to the delivery room. One member of the team connects a blender to oxygen and air sources and attaches an extremely preterm-sized mask to the resuscitation bag. The temperature in the delivery room is increased and a disposable warming pad is activated and placed under several layers of warming blankets under a pre-warmed radiant warmer. The bottom is cut from a closable food storage bag and placed on the blankets. A laryngoscope with a size 0 blade is assembled and checked for a functioning light and a size 2.5-mm endotracheal tube is brought to the resuscitation table. A leader is identified and the team discusses what likely will be required during the resuscitation, including who will be responsible for the airway, monitoring the heart rate, emergent umbilical venous catheterization, and preparation of medications. An additional person is recruited to record all events. The leader identifies herself to the mother and father and explains the anticipated upcoming events.

The baby is delivered, the cord is cut, and the newborn, weighing approximately 2 lbs, is handed to a member of the resuscitation team who places him up to his neck in the polyethylene bag and lays him gently on the pre-warmed towels under the radiant warmer. Bloody amniotic fluid is suctioned from his mouth and nose, his breathing is stimulated by gently rubbing his extremities, and the third person attaches an oximeter probe to the baby's foot. His tone is fairly good and there are labored respiratory efforts. Continuous positive airway pressure (CPAP) is administered by mask. By 30 seconds of age, the heart rate is approximately 70 beats per minute (bpm) and the baby has fewer respiratory efforts. Positive-pressure ventilations are administered with supplemental oxygen, but, despite adjusting of head position and suctioning of the airway, no breath sounds are audible with a stethoscope, the chest is not moving, and the heart rate is not increasing. The trachea is intubated, correct placement is verified with a CO_2 detector, breath sounds are noted to be equal bilaterally, and the 7-cm mark on the tube is noted to be at the baby's lip. Intermittent positive-pressure ventilation with 100% oxygen at approximately 20 to 22 cm H_2O is gently administered. The oximeter begins to register a heart rate greater than 100 bpm and an oxygen saturation in the 70s that is increasing. The baby is 2 minutes old. Breath sounds are audible and slight chest movement is present. As the saturation continues to rise, the oxygen concentration is gradually decreased. By 5 minutes of age, the heart rate is 150 bpm and the saturation is approximately 90% as intermittent positive pressure with 50% oxygen is continued. The peak inflation pressure is decreased to the minimum amount required to achieve a sustained heart rate above 100 bpm, with perceptible chest wall movement. At 10 minutes of age, surfactant is administered down the endotracheal tube. By 15 minutes, the oxygen concentration has been weaned to 25%. The baby is shown to his parents and transported to the nursery in a transport incubator while receiving positive-pressure ventilation.

What will this lesson cover?

In the first 7 lessons, you learned a systematic approach to resuscitating a baby after birth, and how to apply those principles when resuscitating an infant during the first few weeks after birth. The resuscitation steps that you now know so well are aimed at assisting babies to make the transition from a fluid-filled, intrauterine environment to extrauterine life, most at a time that they normally would, but for some reason were unable to do so independently.

When birth occurs before term, there are numerous additional challenges that the fetus must overcome to make this difficult transition. The likelihood that the preterm baby will need your help becomes greater as the degree of prematurity increases. Complications of prematurity and many of the lifelong problems that can be associated with preterm birth are triggered by events that occur just before and during these few transitional minutes. Although the steps of resuscitation you have learned thus far still apply when resuscitating a preterm baby, this lesson focuses on the additional problems associated with preterm birth and highlights actions that you can take to prevent them.

Why are premature babies at higher risk?

Babies who are born before term are at risk for a variety of complications following birth; some of these risk factors may have contributed to them having been born preterm. Premature babies are anatomically and physiologically immature.

- Their thin skin, large surface area relative to body mass, and decreased fat allow them to lose heat easier.

- Their immature tissues may be more easily damaged by excessive oxygen.

- Their weak muscles may make it difficult for them to breathe.

- Their drive to breathe may be decreased due to immaturity of the nervous system.

- Their lungs may be immature and deficient in surfactant, thus making ventilation difficult and their lungs more easily injured by positive-pressure ventilation.

- Their immune systems are immature, thus making it more likely to be born with an infection and to develop infection after birth.

- Fragile capillaries within their developing brains may rupture.

- Their small blood volume makes them more susceptible to the hypovolemic effects of blood loss.

These and other aspects of prematurity should alert you to seek extra help when anticipating the birth of a baby born preterm.

What additional resources do you need?

- *Additional trained personnel*
  The chances that a premature baby will require resuscitation are significantly higher than for a baby born at term. Additional monitoring is required and there may be additional respiratory equipment to be managed. Also, if the baby is significantly preterm, there is a higher likelihood that endotracheal intubation will be needed. Therefore, recruit extra personnel to be present at the birth, including someone skilled in endotracheal intubation.

- *Additional means of maintaining temperature*
  Increase the temperature in the delivery room and preheat the radiant warmer to ensure a warm environment for the baby. If the baby is anticipated to be significantly preterm (for example, less than 28 weeks' gestation), you may want to have a reclosable, food-grade polyethylene bag and a portable warming pad ready, as described in the next section. A transport incubator is helpful for maintaining the baby's temperature during the move to the nursery after resuscitation.

This Neonatal Resuscitation Program (NRP) currently recommends that resuscitation of extremely preterm babies should be accomplished ideally with the capability to administer less than 100% oxygen. However, if a hospital normally transfers high-risk mothers to a higher-level facility, that hospital very rarely will be called upon to resuscitate an extremely preterm baby. These rare cases may occur when transfer of the mother is contraindicated, such as when labor has progressed too far for transfer to be accomplished safely. In such cases, resuscitation using 100% oxygen is acceptable, as research studies have not proven that it is essential to use less than 100% oxygen for the brief period required for resuscitation. Therefore, the following equipment is recommended for the delivery areas of any facility that electively delivers babies at less than approximately 32 weeks' gestation. As further research becomes available, such equipment eventually may be recommended for all hospitals that deliver babies.

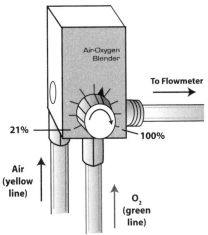

- **Compressed air source**
  You will need a source of compressed air (either wall or compressed gas tank) to mix air with 100% oxygen to achieve an oxygen concentration adjustable between 21% (room air) and 100% oxygen.

- **Oxygen blender (Figure 8.1)**
  An oxygen blender is needed to deliver an oxygen concentration between 21% and 100%. High-pressure hoses run from the oxygen and air sources to the blender, which has a dial that adjusts the gas from 21% to 100% oxygen. An adjustable flowmeter connects to the blender so that flow rates of 0 to 20 L/min of the desired oxygen concentration can be delivered directly to the baby or to the positive-pressure delivery device.

Figure 8.1. Mixing oxygen and air with an oxygen blender. The control knob dials in the desired oxygen concentration

- **Pulse oximeter (Figure 8.2)**
  Oxygen is transported from the lungs to tissues by hemoglobin in the red blood cells. The hemoglobin changes color from blue to red as it carries more oxygen. This change in color can be measured with a pulse oximeter that is attached to a baby's hand or foot. The oximeter gives a reading ranging from 0% to 100% and is useful in determining whether a baby has a satisfactory amount of oxygen in his or her blood.

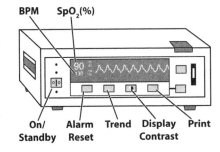

Figure 8.2. Pulse oximeter for measuring the oxyhemoglobin saturation

How do you keep the baby warm?

Premature babies are particularly vulnerable to cold stress. Their larger surface-area-to-body-mass ratio, thin permeable skin, small amount of subcutaneous fat, and limited metabolic response to cold may lead to rapid heat loss and decrease in body temperature. Babies born prematurely should have all steps taken to reduce heat loss, even if they do not initially appear to require resuscitation. Therefore, when a preterm delivery is expected, anticipate that temperature regulation will be challenging and prepare for it.

- *Increase the temperature of the delivery room.* Frequently, delivery rooms and operating rooms are maintained relatively cool for the comfort of the laboring mother and for surgical personnel who must wear multiple layers of protective clothing. When delivery of a preterm baby is anticipated, the temperature of the room should be increased, if possible, for the brief period required for resuscitation and stabilization of the baby. Some facilities have a separate adjacent resuscitation area for the baby. If so, this area should be pre-warmed.

- *Pre-heat the radiant warmer* by turning it on well before the birth.

- *Place a portable warming pad under the layers of towels* that are on the resuscitation table. These pads are commercially available and are warmed only when needed, by activating a chemical reaction within the pad. The pads are designed not to overheat. Follow the manufacturer's recommendation for activation and place the correct side next to the baby.

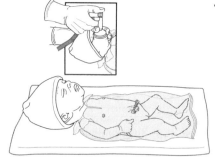

Figure 8.3. Use of a plastic bag for reducing evaporative heat loss

- *If the baby is born at less than 28 weeks' gestation, consider placing him, below the neck, in a reclosable polyethylene bag (Figure 8.3).* Although you learned in Lesson 2 that evaporative heat loss can be decreased by drying the baby immediately following birth, the same purpose can be accomplished by placing the baby's body, below the neck, in a plastic bag, without first drying the skin. This also avoids the stress that may occur with vigorous rubbing and saves the time normally required to change wet linens. The bag can be a standard 1-gallon, food-quality, polyethylene bag purchased in a grocery store. Before the delivery, use scissors to make an opening in the closed end, sufficiently large for the baby's head. Then, after the baby has been placed in the bag, with his head brought through the cut end, and the baby has been appropriately resuscitated, the reclosable end can be closed to minimize further evaporation.

- When the baby is transported to the nursery after resuscitation, *use a pre-warmed transport incubator* to maintain adequate temperature control *en route*.

Note: Rare cases of overheating have been described with use of the plastic-bag technique. Simultaneous use of all these strategies for maintaining temperature control has not been studied. Be sure to monitor the baby's temperature and avoid overheating as well as cooling. The goal should be an axillary temperature of approximately 36.5°C.

Review

(The answers are in the preceding section and at the end of the lesson.)

1. List 5 factors that increase the risk of resuscitation with preterm babies.

   _____

   _____

   _____

   _____

   _____

2. A baby is about to be born at 30 weeks' gestation. What additional resources should you assemble?

   _____

   _____

   _____

   _____

   _____

3. You have turned on the radiant warmer in anticipation of the birth of a baby at 27 weeks' gestation. What else might you consider to help maintain this baby's temperature?

   _____

   _____

   _____

How much oxygen should you use?

You have learned in previous lessons that injury during perinatal transition results from inadequate blood flow and limited oxygen delivery to body tissues, and that restoring these factors are an important goal in resuscitation. However, research at both the cellular and whole-body levels suggests that excessive oxygen, delivered to tissues that have been deprived of perfusion and oxygen, can result in even worse injury. Hyperoxic re-perfusion injury may be a more significant factor for the infant born preterm, because development of tissues during fetal life normally occurs in a relatively low oxygen environment, and the mechanisms that protect the body from oxidant injury have not yet fully developed.

As noted in Lesson 3, research studies so far have been unable to define precisely how quickly a baby who has been deprived of oxygen should be re-oxygenated. When resuscitating babies born at term, the NRP advises using 100% oxygen whenever a baby is cyanotic or whenever positive-pressure ventilation is required. However, when resuscitating a preterm baby, in addition to giving sufficient oxygen to correct the baby's hypoxemic state, you should also be vigilant about avoiding excessive oxygen. To accomplish these goals, you will need an oxygen blender and a pulse oximeter to vary the amount of oxygen being given and to measure the amount of oxygen being absorbed by the baby. This additional equipment is especially recommended if preterm babies born at less than approximately 32 weeks' gestation are delivered electively at your facility. If your facility does not have these resources and there is insufficient time to transfer the mother to another facility, the resources and oxygen management described for a term baby in Lessons 1 through 7 are appropriate to use during resuscitation. (See color Figures F-1, F-2, F-3, and F-4 in the center of the book.)

How do you adjust the oxygen?

The amount of oxygen used during resuscitation is determined by your clinical assessment, the concentration of oxygen delivered, and the reading from a pulse oximeter attached to the baby. During development in utero, a fetus normally has an oxyhemoglobin saturation of approximately 60%. Air-breathing children and adults normally have oxyhemoglobin saturations of 95% to 100%. Observational studies conducted with full-term babies following uncomplicated birth and initiation of air breathing have shown that it may normally take more than 10 minutes for oxyhemoglobin saturations to rise to 90% and that occasional dips to the high 80% range are normal during the first few days of extrauterine life.

Studies have not been conducted to define the optimum oxyhemoglobin saturation for a premature baby during the first few minutes following birth. However, because preterm babies are particularly sensitive to excessive tissue oxygen, long periods of saturations of more than 95% may be too high if a preterm baby is receiving supplemental oxygen. Therefore, several steps are recommended to reduce excessive tissue oxygenation if a very preterm baby is being electively delivered at your facility. These steps become more important as gestational age decreases. Conversely, if your delivery facility does not have resources for diluting oxygen, there is not convincing evidence that a brief period of 100% oxygen during resuscitation will be detrimental.

1. Connect a blender to compressed oxygen and air sources and to the positive-pressure device. It is recommended that you start somewhere between room air (21%) and 100% oxygen so that you can either increase or decrease the concentration as the baby's condition indicates. There are no studies to justify starting at any particular concentration.

2. Attach a pulse oximeter to the baby's foot or hand while the initial steps of resuscitation are being performed. The method of attaching the oximeter sensor will depend on the brand of oximeter. Follow the manufacturer's recommendation.

3. Watch the oximeter for a reliable signal. The oximeter will display both a heart rate and a saturation reading. The heart rate reading should agree with the heart rate that you palpate from the umbilical pulse or hear with a stethoscope. The saturation reading is not reliable until the heart rate reading is accurate. It may take several minutes to achieve reliable readings. If the oximeter continues to fail to display a reading, there may be insufficient cardiac output or the probe may need to be reapplied.

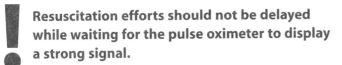

Resuscitation efforts should not be delayed while waiting for the pulse oximeter to display a strong signal.

4. Adjust the oxygen concentration from the blender either up or down to achieve an oxyhemoglobin concentration that gradually increases toward 90%. During the first few minutes, saturations of 70% to 80% may be acceptable, as long as the heart rate is increasing, the baby is being ventilated, and the oxygen saturations are increasing. If saturations are less than 85% and are not increasing, increase the oxygen concentration being delivered from the blender (or increase the amount of positive pressure being delivered if the chest is not moving). Decrease the oxygen concentration as saturations rise above 95%.

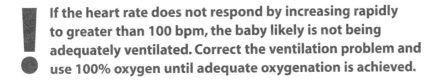

If the heart rate does not respond by increasing rapidly to greater than 100 bpm, the baby likely is not being adequately ventilated. Correct the ventilation problem and use 100% oxygen until adequate oxygenation is achieved.

How do you assist ventilation?

Babies born significantly preterm have immature lungs that may be difficult to ventilate but are also more easily injured with intermittent positive-pressure breaths. If the baby is breathing spontaneously and has a heart rate above 100 bpm, it may be preferable to let him continue to progress through the first few minutes of transition without assistance. However, use the same criteria for assisting ventilation with a preterm baby that you have learned for assisting ventilation with a term baby (see flow diagram). The following are special considerations for assisting ventilation of preterm babies:

Consider giving CPAP. If the baby is breathing spontaneously and has a heart rate above 100 bpm, but appears to have labored respirations or is cyanotic or having low oxygen saturation, administration of continuous positive airway pressure (CPAP) may be helpful. Continuous positive airway pressure is administered by placing the mask of a flow-inflating bag or T-piece resuscitator tightly on the baby's face and adjusting the flow-control valve (Figure 8.4) or positive end-expiratory pressure (PEEP) valve (Figure 8.5) to the desired amount of CPAP. Generally, 4 to 6 cm H_2O is an adequate amount of pressure. *Continuous positive airway pressure cannot be delivered with a self-inflating bag.*

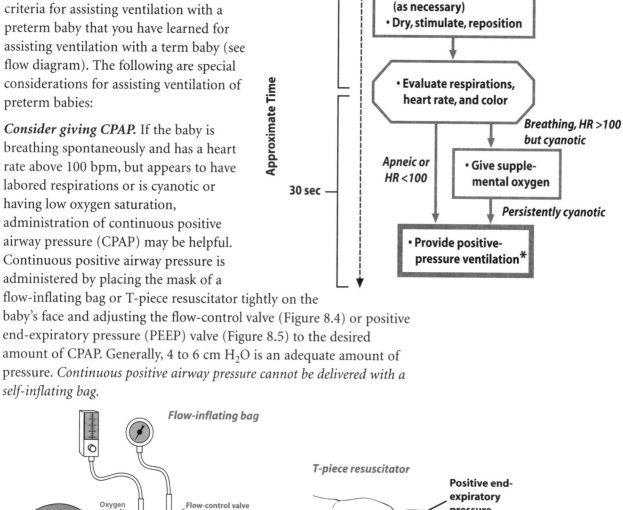

Birth

- Term gestation?
- Clear amniotic fluid?
- Breathing or crying?
- Good muscle tone?

No

30 sec

- Provide warmth
- Position; clear airway* (as necessary)
- Dry, stimulate, reposition

- Evaluate respirations, heart rate, and color

Apneic or HR <100

Breathing, HR >100 but cyanotic

- Give supplemental oxygen

Persistently cyanotic

30 sec

- Provide positive-pressure ventilation*

Approximate Time

Flow-inflating bag

Oxygen Flow-control valve

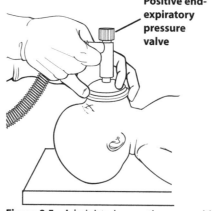

T-piece resuscitator

Positive end-expiratory pressure valve

Figure 8.4. Administering continuous positive airway pressure with a flow-inflating bag

Figure 8.5. Administering continuous positive airway pressure with a T-piece resuscitator

Use the lowest inflation pressure necessary to achieve an adequate response. If intermittent positive-pressure ventilation is required due to apnea, a heart rate less than 100 bpm, or persistent cyanosis, an initial inflation pressure of 20 to 25 cm H_2O is adequate for most preterm infants. If prompt improvement in heart rate or chest movement is not obtained, then higher pressures may be needed. However, be careful to avoid creating excessive chest rise during ventilation of preterm infants immediately after birth, as their lungs are easily injured.

Consider giving surfactant if the baby is significantly preterm. Studies have shown that babies born at less than approximately 30 weeks' gestation benefit from being given surfactant after resuscitation, but while still in the delivery room and even if they have not yet developed significant respiratory distress. However, the indications for and timing of surfactant administration remain controversial. Prophylactic administration of surfactant will be determined by local care practices.

Babies should be fully resuscitated before surfactant is given.

What can you do to decrease the chances of brain injury?

The brains of babies born before approximately 32 weeks' gestation have a very fragile structure called the germinal matrix. The germinal matrix consists of a network of capillaries that are prone to rupture, particularly if the baby is handled too vigorously, if there are rapid changes in blood carbon dioxide (CO_2) or blood pressure, or if anything obstructs venous drainage from the head. A ruptured germinal matrix results in intraventricular hemorrhage that can be associated with lifelong disability. The following precautions could apply to babies of all gestational ages, but are especially important when resuscitating a preterm baby to help avoid intraventricular bleeding:

Handle the baby gently. While this may seem obvious whenever treating any baby, this aspect of care may be forgotten during the stress of a resuscitation when all members of the team are trying to act quickly and effectively.

Avoid placing the baby in a head-down (Trendelenburg) position. The resuscitation table should be flat.

Avoid delivering excessive positive pressure or CPAP. Sufficient pressure to achieve a rise in heart rate and adequate ventilation should be provided, but excessive inflation pressure or too much CPAP can restrict venous return from the head or create a pneumothorax, both of which have been associated with an increased risk of intraventricular hemorrhage.

Use an oximeter and blood gases to adjust ventilation and oxygen concentration gradually and appropriately. Rapid changes in CO_2 result in corresponding changes in cerebral flow, which can increase the risk of bleeding.

Do not give rapid infusions of fluid. If volume expansion becomes necessary (see Lesson 6), avoid giving the infusion too rapidly. Also, avoid giving hypertonic solutions intravenously. If intravenous dextrose is indicated to treat hypoglycemia, try initially to avoid using concentrations greater than approximately 10%.

What special precautions should be taken after a preterm baby has been successfully resuscitated?

Most of the physiologic preparation for a baby to become independent of his or her mother occurs during the last trimester. If a baby is born prematurely, many of these adaptations have not occurred and the preterm baby who has required resuscitation is even more susceptible to the stresses of independent survival. Consider the following precautions when initially managing a premature baby who required resuscitation at birth:

Monitor blood sugar. Babies born preterm have lower glycogen stores than babies born at term. If resuscitation is required, it is more likely that these stores will be depleted quickly. Therefore, preterm babies who require resuscitation are at high risk for developing hypoglycemia.

Monitor the baby for apnea and bradycardia. Respiratory control is often unstable in preterm babies. If oxygen, CO_2, electrolytes, or other metabolic variables become disarranged (as they are more likely to do following resuscitation), the first clinical sign may be apnea followed by bradycardia.

Give an appropriate amount of oxygen and ventilation. Following resuscitation, premature babies continue to be particularly vulnerable to both hypoxemia and hyperoxemia. Continue to monitor pulse oximetry until you are confident that the baby can maintain normal oxygenation while breathing room air. If the baby continues to require positive-pressure ventilation, measure a blood gas to guide the amount of assisted ventilation required.

Give feedings slowly and cautiously while you maintain nutrition intravenously. Premature babies are at risk for developing necrotizing enterocolitis—a life-threatening bowel disease that is more likely to occur if there has been an episode of bowel ischemia. Therefore, premature babies who require resuscitation are at particularly high risk of developing necrotizing enterocolitis. Many neonatologists and gastroenterologists believe that babies at risk for necrotizing enterocolitis should have feedings withheld or introduced slowly and cautiously. Intravenous nutrition may be needed during this time.

Increase suspicion for infection. Preterm babies have immature immune mechanisms, and amnionitis is thought to be a major reason for the onset of preterm labor. Fetal infection may cause perinatal depression at birth, and necessitate resuscitation. If a preterm baby who required resuscitation continues to be symptomatic, consider infection as a cause and the need for antibiotic therapy.

Key Points

1. Preterm babies are at additional risk for requiring resuscitation because of their
   - Excessive heat loss
   - Vulnerability to hyperoxic injury
   - Immature lungs and diminished respiratory drive
   - Immature brains that are prone to bleeding
   - Vulnerability to infection
   - Low blood volume, increasing the implications of blood loss

2. Additional resources needed to prepare for an anticipated preterm birth include
   - Additional trained personnel, including intubation expertise
   - Additional strategies for maintaining temperature
   - Compressed air
   - Oxygen blender
   - Pulse oximetry

3. Premature babies are more vulnerable to hyperoxia; use an oximeter and blender to gradually achieve oxyhemoglobin saturations in the 85% to 95% range during and immediately following resuscitation.

4. When assisting ventilation in preterm babies,
   - Follow the same criteria for initiating positive-pressure ventilation as with term babies.
   - Use the lowest inflation pressure to achieve an adequate response.
   - Consider using CPAP if the baby is breathing spontaneously and has a heart rate above 100 bpm, but is having difficulty such as labored respirations, persistent cyanosis, or low oxygen saturation.
   - Consider giving prophylactic surfactant.

5. Decrease the risk of brain injury by
   - Handling the baby gently
   - Avoiding the Trendelenburg position
   - Avoiding high airway pressures, when possible
   - Adjusting ventilation gradually, based on physical examination, oximetry, and blood gases
   - Avoiding rapid intravenous fluid boluses and hypertonic solutions

6. After resuscitation of a preterm baby,
   - Monitor and control blood sugar.
   - Monitor for apnea, bradycardia, or oxygen desaturations and intervene promptly.
   - Monitor and control oxygenation and ventilation.
   - Consider delaying feeding if perinatal compromise was significant.
   - Increase your suspicion for infection.

Lesson 8 Review

(The answers follow.)

1. List 5 factors that increase the risk of resuscitation with preterm babies.

   _____

   _____

   _____

   _____

   _____

2. A baby is about to be born at 30 weeks' gestation. What additional resources should you assemble?

   _____

   _____

   _____

   _____

   _____

3. You have turned on the radiant warmer in anticipation of the birth of a baby at 27 weeks' gestation. What else might you consider to help maintain this baby's temperature?

   _____

   _____

   _____

4. A baby is delivered at 30 weeks' gestation. He requires positive-pressure ventilation for an initial heart rate of 80 bpm, despite tactile stimulation. He responds quickly with rising heart rate and spontaneous respirations. At 2 minutes of age, he is breathing, has a heart rate of 140 bpm, and is receiving continuous positive airway pressure with a flow-inflating mask and 50% oxygen. You have attached an oximeter that is now reading 85% and is increasing. You should (increase the oxygen concentration) (decrease the oxygen concentration) (leave the oxygen concentration the same).

5. Continuous positive airway pressure may be given with a (choose as many as are correct):
   A. Self-inflating bag
   B. Flow-inflating bag
   C. T-piece resuscitator

Lesson 8 Review — *continued*

6. To decrease the chance of brain hemorrhage, the best position is (table flat) (head down).

7. Intravenous fluids should be given (rapidly) (slowly) to preterm babies.

8. List 3 precautions when managing a preterm baby who has required resuscitation.

   _____

   _____

   _____

Answers to Questions

1. Risk factors include
   - **Lose heat easily**
   - **Tissues easily damaged from excess oxygen**
   - **Weak muscles, making it difficult to breathe**
   - **Lungs deficient in surfactant**
   - **Immature immune systems**
   - **Fragile capillaries in the brain**
   - **Small blood volume**

2. Additional resources include
   - **Additional personnel**
   - **Additional means to control temperature**
   - **Compressed air**
   - **Oxygen blender**
   - **Oximeter**

3. Additional considerations include
   - **Increase temperature of delivery room.**
   - **Activate portable heating pad.**
   - **Prepare plastic bag.**
   - **Prepare a transport incubator.**

4. **Leave the oxygen concentration the same.**

5. Continuous positive airway pressure may be given with a **flow-inflating bag** or a **T-piece resuscitator.**

6. The best position is **table flat.**

7. Intravenous fluids should be given **slowly.**

8. After resuscitation,
   - **Check blood sugar.**
   - **Monitor for apnea.**
   - **Control oxygenation.**
   - **Consider delaying feedings.**
   - **Increase suspicion for infection.**

Ethics and Care at the End of Life

In Lesson 9 you will learn

- **The ethical principles associated with starting and stopping neonatal resuscitation**

- **How to communicate with parents and to involve them in ethical decision making**

- **When it may be appropriate to withhold resuscitation**

- **What to do when the prognosis is uncertain**

- **How long to continue resuscitation attempts when the baby does not respond**

- **What to do when a baby dies**

- **How to help parents through the grieving process**

- **How to help staff through the grieving process**

Notes: Although this lesson is directed at the resuscitation team member who guides medical decision making, all members of the team should understand the reasoning behind the decisions. As much as possible, there should be unified support of the parents during their very personal period of crisis. This lesson refers to "parents," although it is recognized that sometimes the mother or father is alone during the crisis and, other times, support will be available through extended family or significant others. This lesson is applicable to health care professionals who participate in all levels of neonatal resuscitation plus professionals providing care to families who have experienced a neonatal death.

Mortality and morbidity data by gestational age may be found at the Neonatal Resuscitation Program (NRP) Web site (http://www.aap.org/nrp).

It is recognized that the recommendations made in this lesson are determined, to an extent, by the cultural context of the United States and will require adaptation to other cultures and countries. It also is recognized that the recommendations are determined by the current, and not necessarily future, outcomes experience.

Case 9.
Care of a baby who could not be resuscitated

A gravida 3 woman at 23 weeks' gestation is admitted to the obstetrics floor of a rural community hospital with contractions, fever, and ruptured membranes. Gestation had been estimated by serial first- and second-trimester ultrasounds. The obstetrician asks you to join her in talking with the parents about the implications of a delivery at this early gestation. Before the meeting, the 2 of you discuss your regional mortality statistics over the past 5 years and the national information about long-term morbidity of survivors following a birth at 23 weeks' gestation and probable chorioamnionitis. The obstetrician advises against tocolysis because of suspected chorioamnionitis, and states that labor has progressed too far to try to transport the mother. You both enter the mother's room, introduce yourselves, and suggest that visitors may want to move to the waiting room while you talk with both parents, unless the parents prefer that they stay. The television is turned off and you both sit in chairs by the mother's bed.

The obstetrician describes the obstetric care plan. You explain the implications of extremely preterm birth with overlying chorioamnionitis, including the mortality and morbidity statistics and some of the expectations associated with neonatal intensive care. You describe the resuscitation team that will be available for the delivery, what procedures might be required to assist the baby's survival, and that some parents might elect not to attempt resuscitation in view of the risks involved for the likely outcome. The parents respond that they "want everything done if there is any chance that our baby can live."

Over the next hour, labor progresses, delivery becomes imminent, and the neonatal transport team at the regional medical center is alerted. Appropriate preparations of equipment and staff are made for an extremely preterm delivery. When the baby is presented to the neonatal team, he has thin gelatinous skin, no tone, and minimal respiratory efforts. A bad odor suggests chorioamnionitis. The initial steps and positive-pressure ventilation by mask are administered, and a heart rate of approximately 40 beats per minute (bpm) is detected. The trachea is intubated and positive-pressure ventilation via the endotracheal tube is continued. However, despite further resuscitation steps, the heart rate gradually falls and the pediatrician explains to the parents that resuscitation has been unsuccessful. The endotracheal tube is removed, the baby is wrapped in a clean blanket, and the parents are asked if they would like to hold him. The parents do so and a member of the team remains with them to offer support. A picture is taken and given to the parents. The baby is pronounced dead when no signs of life remain.

Later that day, a member of the nursery team returns to the parents' room, expresses condolences, answers questions about the resuscitation, and asks the parents about an autopsy. The next day a funeral home is identified. About 1 month later, a member of the nursery team contacts the parents, offering to schedule an office visit to discuss autopsy results and implications and problems the parents and siblings may be having adjusting to their loss, and to answer any questions that may remain about their son's death.

What ethical principles apply to neonatal resuscitation?

The ethical principles of neonatal resuscitation are no different from those followed in resuscitating an older child or adult. Common ethical principles that apply to all medical care include respecting an individual's rights of freedom and liberty to make changes that affect his or her life (autonomy), acting so as to benefit others (beneficence), avoiding harming people unnecessarily (nonmaleficence), and treating people truthfully and fairly (justice). These principles underlie why we ask patients for informed consent before proceeding with treatment. Exceptions to this rule include life-threatening medical emergencies and when patients are not competent to make their own decisions. Neonatal resuscitation is a medical treatment often complicated by both of these exceptions.

Unlike adults, infants cannot make decisions for themselves and cannot express their desires. A surrogate decision maker must be identified to assume the responsibility of guarding the infant's best interests. Parents are generally considered to be the best surrogate decision makers for their own infants. For parents to fulfill this role responsibly, they need relevant, accurate, and honest information about the risks and benefits of each treatment option. In addition, they must have adequate time to thoughtfully consider each option, ask additional questions, and seek other opinions. Unfortunately, the need for resuscitation is often an unexpected emergency with little opportunity to achieve fully informed consent before proceeding. Even when you have the opportunity to meet with parents, uncertainty about the extent of congenital anomalies, the actual gestational age, the likelihood of survival, and the potential for severe disabilities may make it difficult for parents to decide before the delivery what is in their baby's best interest. In rare cases, the health care team may conclude that a decision made by a parent is not reasonable and is not in the baby's best interest.

The NRP endorses the following statement from the American Medical Association (AMA) Code of Medical Ethics:

> The primary consideration for decisions regarding life-sustaining treatment for seriously ill newborns should be what is best for the newborn. Factors that should be weighed are as follows:
>
> 1. The chance that the therapy will succeed
> 2. The risks involved with treatment and nontreatment
> 3. The degree to which the therapy, if successful, will extend life
> 4. The pain and discomfort associated with the therapy
> 5. The anticipated quality of life for the newborn with and without treatment
>
> (American Medical Association, Council on Ethical and Judicial Affairs. *Code of Medical Ethics: Current Opinions with Annotations*, 2004–2005 ed. Chicago, IL: American Medical Association; 2002:92 [sect 2.215])

What laws apply to neonatal resuscitation?

There is no United States federal law mandating delivery room resuscitation in all circumstances. There may be laws in your area that apply to the care of newborns in the delivery room. Health care providers should be aware of the laws in the areas that they practice. If you are uncertain about the laws in your area, you should consult your hospital ethics committee or attorney. In most circumstances, it is ethically and legally acceptable to withhold or withdraw resuscitation efforts if the parents and health professionals agree that further medical intervention would be futile, would merely prolong dying, or would not offer sufficient benefit to justify the burdens imposed.

What role should parents play in decisions about resuscitation?

Parents have the primary role in determining the goals of care delivered to their newborn. However, informed consent should be based on complete and reliable information, and this may not be available until after delivery and perhaps not until several hours after birth.

 Caution: Be careful not to make rigid promises about withholding or initiating resuscitation before information needed to make that decision is available.

Are there situations in which it is ethical not to initiate resuscitation?

The delivery of extremely immature babies and those with severe congenital anomalies frequently raises questions about the initiation of resuscitation. Although the survival rate for babies born between 22 and 25 weeks' gestation increases with each additional week of gestation, the incidence of moderate or severe neurodevelopmental disability among survivors is high. Where gestation, birth weight, and/or congenital anomalies are associated with almost certain early death, and unacceptably high morbidity is likely among the rare survivors, resuscitation is not indicated, although exceptions may be appropriate in specific cases to comply with parental request. Examples may include the following:

- Newborns with a confirmed gestational age of less than 23 weeks or a birth weight of less than 400 g.
- Anencephaly
- Confirmed Trisomy 13 or Trisomy 18 syndrome

In conditions associated with uncertain prognosis, where there is borderline survival and a relatively high rate of morbidity, and where the burden to the child is high, some parents will request that no attempt be made to resuscitate the baby. An example may include a baby born at 23 to 24 weeks' gestation. In such cases, the parents' views on either initiating or withholding resuscitation should be supported.

These recommendations must be interpreted according to current local outcomes and parental desires. Given the uncertainty of gestational age and birth weight predictions, be cautious about making unalterable decisions about resuscitative efforts before the baby is born. When counseling parents, advise them that decisions made about neonatal management before birth may need to be modified in the delivery room, depending on the condition of the baby at birth and the postnatal gestational age assessment.

Unless conception occurred via in vitro fertilization, techniques used for obstetrical dating are accurate only to ± 1 to 2 weeks, and estimates of fetal weight are accurate only to ± 15% to 20%. Even small discrepancies of 1 or 2 weeks in gestational age or 100 to 200 g in birth weight may have implications for survival and long-term morbidity. Also, fetal weight can be misleading if there has been growth restriction. These uncertainties underscore the importance of not making firm commitments about withholding resuscitation until you have the opportunity to examine the baby after birth.

Are there times when you should resuscitate a baby against parental wishes?

Although parents generally are considered the best surrogate decision makers for their own children, health care professionals have a legal and an ethical obligation to provide appropriate care for the infant based on current medical information and their clinical assessment. In conditions associated with a high rate of survival and an acceptable risk of morbidity, resuscitation is nearly always indicated. When the health care team is unable to reach agreement with the parents on a reasonable treatment strategy, it may become necessary to consult the hospital ethics committee or legal counsel. If there is not enough time to consult additional resources, and the responsible physician concludes that the parents' decision is not in the best interest of the child, it is appropriate to resuscitate the infant over the parents' objection. Accurate documentation of the discussions with the parents, as well as documentation of the basis for the decision, is essential.

What discussions should be held with parents prior to a very high-risk birth?

Meeting with parents prior to a very high-risk birth is important for both the parents and the neonatal care providers. Both the obstetrical provider and the provider who will care for the baby after birth should talk with the parents. Studies have shown that obstetrical and neonatal perspectives are often different. If possible, such differences should be discussed prior to meeting with the parents so that the information presented is consistent. Sometimes, such as when the woman is in active labor, it may seem as if there is inadequate time for such discussions. Nevertheless, the meeting should not be postponed. Follow-up meetings can take place if the situation changes over subsequent hours and days.

What should you say when you meet with parents for prenatal counseling before a high-risk birth?

Prenatal discussions provide an opportunity to begin establishing a trusting relationship, provide important information, establish realistic goals, and assist parents in making informed decisions for their baby. If it is impractical to meet the parents with a member of the obstetrical team, obtain a complete history before the meeting and review the obstetrical management plan during the meeting to provide consistent and coordinated care. You should be knowledgeable about short- and long-term outcome data for babies born at extremely premature gestations or with congenital anomalies, both nationally and at your own institution. If necessary, consult with specialists at your regional referral center to obtain up-to-date information. If possible, meet with the parents before the mother has received medications that might make it difficult for her to understand or remember your conversation, and before the final stages of labor.

Before meeting with the parents, check with the mother's nurse to make sure it is a good time for a discussion. If possible, have the nurse attend the meeting. If a translator is necessary, use a hospital-trained and certified medical translator, not a relative of the patient, and use simple and direct phrases to ensure accurate transmittal of information. It is best if you sit down during the meeting to make eye contact at the same level and to avoid the impression of being in a hurry. Use of clear, simple language, without medical abbreviations or jargon, is especially important. Stop talking when the mother is having a contraction or if a procedure, such as vital signs, needs to be performed during the meeting. Resume the discussion when she is again able to concentrate on the information you are providing.

The following issues may be covered:

- Explain your assessment of the baby's chances of survival and possible disability based on regional and national statistics. Be as accurate as possible, avoiding excessively negative or unrealistically positive prognoses.

- If the baby's viability is thought to be marginal, and palliative or "comfort-care-only" treatment may be an acceptable option, do not avoid this issue. The discussion will be difficult for both you and the parents, but it is important that each of you understands the others' perspectives. If the options are discussed, most parents will quickly make clear what they want you to do. You can assure them that you will make every effort to support their wishes, but it is also important to advise them that decisions made about neonatal management before birth may need to be modified in the delivery room depending on the baby's condition at birth, the postnatal gestational age assessment, and the baby's response to resuscitative measures.

- If palliative or comfort care treatment is agreed upon (subject to confirmation of the baby's status as described above), assure the parents that care will focus on preventing or relieving pain and suffering. Explain that, in this case, the baby will die, but the timing could be minutes to hours after birth. In a culturally sensitive manner, discuss ways in which the family might participate, and allow them to make additional suggestions/requests.

- Explain where the resuscitation will occur, and who will be in the delivery room and what their roles will be. The events will likely be very different than the private birth they had originally imagined.

- Offer to give the mother and father (or support person) time alone to discuss what you have told them. Some parents may want to consult with other family members or clergy. Then make a return visit to confirm both their understanding of what may occur and your understanding of their wishes.

After you meet with the parents, document a summary of your conversation in the mother's chart.

Review what you discussed with the obstetrical care providers and the other members of your nursery's resuscitation team. *If it was decided that resuscitation would not be initiated, ensure that all members of your team, including on-call personnel and the obstetric care providers, are informed and in agreement with this decision.* If disagreements occur, discuss them in advance and consult additional professionals if necessary.

What should you do if you are uncertain about the chances of survival or serious disability after examining the baby immediately after birth?

If parents are uncertain how to proceed, or your examination suggests that the prenatal assessment of gestational age was incorrect, initial resuscitation and provision of life support allows you additional time to gather more complete clinical information and permits more time to review the situation with the parents. Once the parents and physicians have had an opportunity to further evaluate additional clinical information, they may decide to discontinue critical care interventions and institute comfort care measures. It should be noted that, although there is no ethical distinction between withholding and withdrawing support, many people find the latter more difficult. Nevertheless, resuscitation followed by withdrawal permits time for collecting more prognostic information. This approach also may be preferable for many parents, as they feel more comfortable that an effort was made. You should avoid a scenario where an initial decision is made not to resuscitate and then aggressive resuscitation is initiated many minutes after delivery due to a change of plan. If the newborn survives this delayed resuscitation, the risk of serious disability may increase.

You have followed the resuscitation recommendations and the baby is not responding. How long should you continue?

If there is no heart rate after 10 minutes of complete and adequate resuscitation efforts, and there is no evidence of other causes of newborn compromise, discontinuation of resuscitation efforts may be appropriate. Current data indicate that, after 10 minutes of asystole, newborns are very unlikely to survive, or the rare survivor is likely to survive with severe disability.

> ⚠️ **Discontinuation of resuscitation efforts after 10 minutes of asystole does not necessarily mean that only 10 minutes will have elapsed from the time of birth. More than 10 minutes may have been required to assess the baby and to optimize the resuscitation efforts.**

There may be other situations where, after complete and adequate resuscitation efforts, discontinuation of resuscitation may be appropriate. However, studies have not been performed from which definitive recommendations can be made.

Once you have resuscitated a baby, are you obligated to continue life support?

In addition to the guideline of discontinuing resuscitation after 10 minutes of asystole, there is also no obligation to continue life support if it is the judgment of experienced clinicians that such support would not be in the best interest of the baby or would serve no useful purpose (ie, would be futile). In the case of withdrawal of critical care interventions and institution of comfort care, the parents should also be in agreement with this judgment.

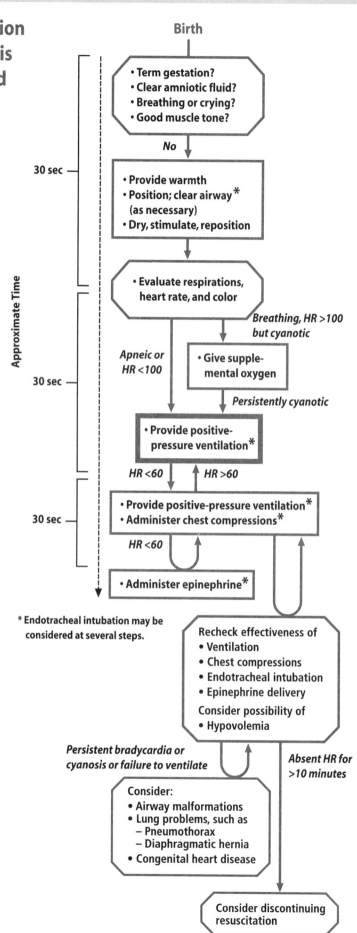

How do you tell the parents that their baby has died or is dying?

As soon as possible, sit down with the mother and the father (or another support person) to tell them that their baby has died (or is dying). There are no words that will make this conversation any less painful. Do not use euphemisms, such as, "Your baby has passed." Refer to the baby by name if the parents have already chosen one or by the correct gender if a name has not yet been chosen. Tell them that you are very sorry, but the baby was too ill or too premature to survive. Reassure them that they are good and loving parents and they did not cause the problem. Your role is to support the parents by giving clear and honest information in a supportive and caring manner. Families have described comments made by some providers that were more upsetting than comforting. Be careful ***not*** to say the following:

- "It was for the best" or "It was meant to be."
- "You can have more children."
- "At least it was a baby and you didn't really have time to get to know her."

How do you take care of a baby that is dying or has died?

The most important goal is to provide humane and compassionate care. Offer to bring the baby to the mother and father to hold. Silence the alarms on monitors and medical equipment before removing them. Remove any unnecessary tubes, tape, monitors, or medical equipment and gently clean the baby's mouth and face. Wrap the baby in a clean blanket. Prepare the parents for what they may see, feel, and hear when they hold their baby, including the possibility of gasping respirations, color changes, persistent heart beat, and continuing movements. If the baby has obvious congenital anomalies, briefly explain to the parents what they will see. Help them look beyond any deformities by pointing out a good or memorable feature.

It is best to allow the parents private time with the baby in a comfortable environment, but a provider should check at intervals to see if anything is needed. The baby's chest should be auscultated intermittently for at least 60 seconds, as a very slow heart rate may persist for hours. Disturbing noises such as phone calls, pagers, monitor alarms, and staff conversations should be minimized. When the parents are ready for you to take the baby, the baby should be taken to a designated, private location until ready to be transported to the morgue.

It is very helpful to understand the cultural and religious expectations surrounding death in the community that you serve. Some families grieve quietly while others are more demonstrative; however, all modes are acceptable and should be accommodated. Some parents may prefer to be alone, while others may want their extended family, friends, community members, and/or clergy to be with them. Families may request to take their baby to a hospital chapel or a more peaceful setting outside, or may ask for help with arrangements for blessings or rites for their dead or dying baby. You should be as flexible as you can in responding to their wishes.

What follow-up arrangements should be planned for the parents?

Before the parents leave the hospital, make sure you have contact information for them, and provide them with details about how to contact the attending physician, bereavement professionals, and, if available, a perinatal loss support group. Plan to meet to review autopsy results and to answer questions that may remain. It is important to involve the family's primary care physicians so they can provide additional support for the mother, father, and surviving siblings. The attending physician may want to schedule a follow-up appointment to answer any unresolved questions, review results of studies pending at the time of death or autopsy results, and assess the family's needs. Some hospitals sponsor parent-to-parent support groups and plan an annual memorial service, bringing together families who have suffered a perinatal loss. Recognize that some families may not want any additional contact from the hospital staff. This desire must be respected. Unexpected communications, such as a quality assurance survey from the hospital, or newsletters about baby care, may be an unwanted reminder of the family's loss.

How do you support the staff in the nursery after a perinatal death?

Staff members who participated in the care of the baby and family also need support. They will have feelings of sadness and also may be feeling anger and guilt. Consider holding a debriefing session shortly after the baby's death so you can openly discuss questions and feelings in a professional, supportive, and nonjudgmental forum. However, speculation based on secondhand information should be avoided in such meetings, and questions and issues regarding care decisions and actions should be discussed only in a qualified peer review session and according to hospital policy for such sessions.

Key Points

1. The ethical principles regarding the resuscitation of a newborn should be no different from those followed in resuscitating an older child or adult.

2. Ethical and current national legal principles do not mandate attempted resuscitation in all circumstances, and withdrawal of critical care interventions and institution of comfort care are considered acceptable if there is agreement by health professionals and the parents that further resuscitation efforts would be futile, would merely prolong dying, or would not offer sufficient benefit to justify the burdens imposed.

3. Parents are considered to be the appropriate surrogate decision makers for their own infants. For parents to fulfill this role responsibly, they must be given relevant and accurate information about the risks and benefits of each treatment option.

4. Where gestation, birth weight, and/or congenital anomalies are associated with almost certain early death, or unacceptably high morbidity is likely among the rare survivors, resuscitation is not indicated, although exceptions may be reasonable to comply with parental wishes.

5. In conditions associated with uncertain prognosis, where there is borderline survival and a high rate of morbidity, and where the burden to the child is high, parental desires regarding initiation of resuscitation should be supported.

6. Unless conception occurred via in vitro fertilization, techniques used for obstetrical dating are accurate only to ± 1 to 2 weeks. When counseling parents about the births of babies born at the extremes of prematurity, advise them that decisions made about neonatal management before birth may need to be modified in the delivery room, depending on the condition of the baby at birth and the postnatal gestational age assessment.

7. Discontinuation of resuscitation efforts may be appropriate after 10 minutes of absent heart rate following complete and adequate resuscitation efforts.

Lesson 9 Review

(The answers follow.)

1. The 4 common principles of medical ethics are

   • _____

   • _____

   • _____

   • _____

2. Parents are generally considered to be the best "surrogate" decision makers for their own newborns. (True/False)

3. The parents of a baby about to be born at 23 weeks' gestation have requested that if there is any possibility of brain damage, they do not want any attempt made to resuscitate their baby. Which of the following may be appropriate? (Select as many as appropriate.)
   a. Support their wishes and promise to give "comfort care only" to the baby after birth.
   b. Tell them that you will try to support their decision, but must wait until after you examine the baby after birth to determine what you will do.
   c. Tell them that all medical decisions regarding resuscitation are made by the medical team and the physician-in-charge.
   d. Try to convince them to change their mind.

4. You have been asked to be present for the impending birth of a baby known from prenatal ultrasound and laboratory assessments to have major congenital malformations. List 4 issues that should be covered when you meet the parents.

   • _____

   • _____

   • _____

   • _____

Lesson 9 Review — *continued*

5. A mother enters the delivery suite in active labor at 34 weeks' gestation after having had no prenatal care. She proceeds to deliver a liveborn baby with major malformations that appear to be consistent with Trisomy 18 syndrome. An attempt to resuscitate the baby in an adjacent room is unsuccessful. Which of the following is the most appropriate action?
   a. Explain the situation to the parents and ask them if they would like to hold the baby.
   b. Take the baby away from the area, tell the parents that she was stillborn, and tell them that it would be best if they did not see her.
   c. Tell the parents that she had a major malformation and it "was for the best" that she died because she would have been "disabled anyway."

6. Which of the following is (are) appropriate to say to parents whose baby just died after an unsuccessful resuscitation?
   a. "I'm sorry, we tried to resuscitate your baby, but the resuscitation was unsuccessful and your baby died."
   b. "This is a terrible tragedy, but in view of the malformations, it was meant to be."
   c. "I'm so sorry that your baby died. She is a beautiful baby."
   d. "Fortunately, you are both young and can have another baby."

Lesson 9 Answers to Questions

1. The 4 principles are
   - Respect individual's rights of freedom and liberty to make choices that affect his or her life *(autonomy)*.
   - Act so as to benefit others *(beneficence)*.
   - Avoid harming people unjustifiably *(nonmaleficence)*.
   - Treat people truthfully and fairly *(justice)*.

2. True.

3. b. Tell them that you will try to support their decision, but must wait until you examine the baby after birth to determine what you will do.

4. Any of the following:
   - Review the current obstetrical plans and expectations.
   - Explain who will be present and their respective roles.
   - Explain the statistics and your assessment of the baby's chances for survival and possible disability.
   - Determine the parents' wishes and expectations.
   - Inform the parents that decisions may need to be modified after you can examine the baby.

5. a. Explain the situation to the parents and ask them if they would like to hold the baby.

6. Either or both of the following are appropriate:
   a. "I'm sorry, we tried to resuscitate your baby, but the resuscitation was unsuccessful and your baby died."
   c. "I'm so sorry that your baby died. She is a beautiful baby."

Megacode Assessment Form (Basic)

Learner:	
Evaluator:	Date:
Lessons completed: 1–4	PASS _____ REEVALUATE _____

Scoring: 0 = Not Done   1 = Done incorrectly, incompletely, or out of order   2 = Done correctly in order
- Student <u>must</u> perform each of the 5 **bold** items correctly.
- Scenario must include "Heart rate remains <100 beats per minute (bpm) and no chest movement" to allow demonstration of corrective action (Lesson 3).
- Scenario must include "Heart rate <60 bpm despite positive-pressure ventilation" to demonstrate chest compressions.
- Learner must demonstrate ventilation **and** chest compressions.
- Scenario with meconium-stained fluid is optional.

Lesson	Item	0	1	2
1	**Checks Bag, Mask, and Oxygen Supply**			
	Asks 4 Assessment Questions (Term? Meconium? Breathing? Tone?)			
2	(optional) If meconium is present, determines if endotracheal suction is indicated			
	Positions head, suctions mouth then nose			
	Dries, removes wet towels, and repositions			
	Requests description of breathing, heart rate, and color			
3	**Indicates need for positive-pressure ventilation** (Apnea, heart rate <100 bpm, central cyanosis despite O$_2$)			
	Provides positive-pressure ventilation correctly (40-60 breaths/min)			
	Checks for improvement in heart rate (*Instructor note:* Heart rate does NOT improve.)			
	Takes corrective action when heart rate not rising and chest not moving (Reapply mask, lift jaw forward, reposition head, check secretions, open mouth, increase pressure if necessary.)			
	Reevaluates heart rate (*Instructor note:* Heart rate must remain <60 bpm.)			
4	Identifies need to start chest compressions (Heart rate <60 bpm despite 30 seconds of effective positive-pressure ventilation)			
	Demonstrates correct compression technique (Assess correct finger or thumb placement, compress one third of the anterior-posterior diameter of the chest.)			
	Demonstrates correct rate and coordination with ventilation (Ask student and assistant to switch positions.)			
Closure	Continues/discontinues positive-pressure ventilation appropriately or weans free-flow oxygen			
	Student's Score Subtotals			
	Performed all 5 bold items correctly? Y N Reevaluate			
	Student's Total Score (add subtotals) Maximum score: 30 pts with meconium 28 pts without meconium			
	Minimum passing score: 24 pts with meconium 22 pts without meconium	Pass Reevaluate		

Megacode Assessment Form (Advanced)

Learner:

Evaluator:

Lessons completed: 1–4   5   6

Date:

PASS _____   REEVALUATE _____

Scoring: 0 = Not Done   1 = Done incorrectly, incompletely, or out of order   2 = Done correctly in order
- Student <u>must</u> perform each of the 5 **bold** items correctly.
- Scenario must include required items from each lesson that the student has completed.
- All students must complete Lessons 1-4 and Closure.
- Students taking Lesson 6 must prepare and insert or assist with umbilical venous catheter placement and administer medication (if appropriate to learner's role/scope of practice). These skills are not scored, and are not considered when computing the student's score. However, the instructor may decide if the student needs additional feedback and instruction on these skills.
- Lessons 7 through 9 skills and concepts may be included on Megacode. These skills are not scored, and are not considered when computing the student's score. However, the instructor may decide if the student needs additional feedback and instruction on these skills.

Lesson	Possible Points (circle)	Item	0	1	2
1	2	**Checks Bag, Mask, and Oxygen Supply**			
	2	Asks 4 Assessment Questions (Term? Meconium? Breathing? Tone?)			
2	2 optional	(optional) If meconium, determines if endotracheal suction is indicated			
	2	Positions head, suctions mouth then nose			
	2	Dries, removes wet towels, and repositions			
	2	Requests description of breathing, heart rate, and color			
3	2	**Indicates need for positive-pressure ventilation** (Apnea, heart rate <100 beats per minute [bpm], central cyanosis despite O$_2$)			
	2	**Provides positive-pressure ventilation correctly** (40-60 breaths/min)			
	2	Checks for improvement in heart rate (*Instructor note:* Heart rate does NOT improve.)			
	2	**Takes corrective action when heart rate not rising and chest not moving** (Reapply mask, lift jaw forward, reposition head, check secretions, open mouth, increase pressure if necessary.)			
	2	Reevaluates heart rate (*Instructor note:* Heart rate must remain <60 bpm.)			
4	2	Identifies need to start chest compressions (Heart rate <60 bpm despite 30 seconds of effective positive-pressure ventilation)			
	2	**Demonstrates correct compression technique** (Assess correct finger or thumb placement, compress one third of the anterior-posterior diameter of the chest.)			
	2	Demonstrates correct rate and coordination with ventilation (Ask student and assistant to switch positions.)			
5	2	Identifies need for intubation			
	2	Intubates or assists intubation correctly			
6	2	Identifies need for epinephrine (Heart rate <60 bpm despite positive-pressure ventilation and compressions)			
	No score	Prepares correct dose of epinephrine in syringe (0.1-0.3 mL/kg IV or 0.3-1.0 mL/kg ET)	No score		
		Prepares umbilical venous catheter for insertion			
		Inserts umbilical venous catheter			
		Administers epinephrine via umbilical venous catheter and/or endotracheal tube			
	2 optional	(optional) Identifies need for volume administration			
Closure	2	Continues/discontinues positive-pressure ventilation appropriately or weans free-flow oxygen			
	_____ X .85	Total of all circled points (38 points maximum) Multiply total by .85 = minimum acceptable passing score			

Student's Score Subtotals		
Student's Total Score (add subtotals)		
Performed all 5 bold items correctly?	Y N	Reevaluate
Student attained minimum passing score?	Y	Pass
	N	Reevaluate

Appendix

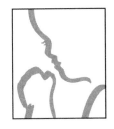

2005 American Heart Association (AHA) Guidelines for Cardiopulmonary Resuscitation (CPR) and Emergency Cardiovascular Care (ECC) of Pediatric and Neonatal Patients: Neonatal Resuscitation Guidelines

American Heart Association, American Academy of Pediatrics

The authors have indicated they have no financial relationships relevant to this article to disclose.

THE FOLLOWING GUIDELINES are intended for practitioners responsible for resuscitating neonates. They apply primarily to neonates undergoing transition from intrauterine to extrauterine life. The recommendations are also applicable to neonates who have completed perinatal transition and require resuscitation during the first few weeks to months following birth. Practitioners who resuscitate infants at birth or at any time during the initial hospital admission should consider following these guidelines. The terms newborn and neonate are intended to apply to any infant during the initial hospitalization. The term newly born is intended to apply specifically to an infant at the time of birth.

Approximately 10% of newborns require some assistance to begin breathing at birth. Approximately 1% require extensive resuscitative measures. Although the vast majority of newly born infants do not require intervention to make the transition from intrauterine to extrauterine life, because of the large number of births, a sizable number will require some degree of resuscitation.

Those newly born infants who do not require resuscitation can generally be identified by a rapid assessment of the following 4 characteristics:

- Was the infant born after a full-term gestation?

- Is the amniotic fluid clear of meconium and evidence of infection?

- Is the infant breathing or crying?

- Does the infant have good muscle tone?

If the answer to all 4 of these questions is "yes," the infant does not need resuscitation and should not be separated from the mother. The infant can be dried, placed directly on the mother's chest, and covered with dry linen to maintain temperature. Observation of breathing, activity, and color should be ongoing.

If the answer to any of these assessment questions is "no," there is general agreement that the infant should receive 1 or more of the following 4 categories of action in sequence:

www.pediatrics.org/cgi/doi/10.1542/peds.2006-0349

doi:10.1542/peds.2006-0349

This report was published in *Circulation*. 2005;112:IV-188–IV-195.

©2005 by the American Heart Association

Key Words
resuscitation, neonatal resuscitation, pediatric advance life support

Abbreviations
LOE—level of evidence
bpm— beats per minute
LMA—laryngeal mask airway
IV—intravenous

Accepted for publication Jan 23, 2006

PEDIATRICS (ISSN Numbers: Print, 0031-4005; Online, 1098-4275). Copyright © 2006 by the American Academy of Pediatrics

A. Initial steps in stabilization (provide warmth, position, clear airway, dry, stimulate, reposition)

B. Ventilation

C. Chest compressions

D. Administration of epinephrine and/or volume expansion

The decision to progress from one category to the next is determined by the simultaneous assessment of 3 vital signs: respirations, heart rate, and color. Approximately 30 seconds is allotted to complete each step, reevaluate, and decide whether to progress to the next step (see Fig 1).

ANTICIPATION OF RESUSCITATION NEED

Anticipation, adequate preparation, accurate evaluation, and prompt initiation of support are critical for successful neonatal resuscitation. At every delivery there should be at least 1 person whose primary responsibility is the newly born. This person must be capable of initiating resuscitation, including administration of positive-pressure ventilation and chest compressions. Either that person or someone else who is immediately available should have the skills required to perform a complete resuscitation, including endotracheal intubation and administration of medications.[1]

With careful consideration of risk factors, the majority of newborns who will need resuscitation can be identified before birth. If the possible need for resuscitation is anticipated, additional skilled personnel should be recruited and the necessary equipment prepared. If a preterm delivery (<37 weeks of gestation) is expected, special preparations will be required. Preterm infants have immature lungs that may be more difficult to ventilate and are also more vulnerable to injury by positive-pressure ventilation. Preterm infants also have immature blood vessels in the brain that are prone to hemorrhage; thin skin and a large surface area, which contribute to rapid heat loss; increased susceptibility to infection; and increased risk of hypovolemic shock caused by small blood volume.

INITIAL STEPS

The initial steps of resuscitation are to provide warmth by placing the infant under a radiant heat source, position the head in a "sniffing" position to open the airway, clear the airway with a bulb syringe or suction catheter, and dry the infant and stimulate breathing. Recent studies have examined several aspects of these initial steps. These studies are summarized below.

TEMPERATURE CONTROL

Very low birth weight (<1500 g) preterm infants are likely to become hypothermic despite the use of traditional techniques for decreasing heat loss (level of evidence [LOE] 5).[2] For this reason it is recommended that additional warming techniques be used, such as covering the infant in plastic wrapping (food-grade, heat-resistant plastic) and placing him or her under radiant heat (Class IIa; LOE 2[3,4]; LOE 4[5,6]; LOE 5[7]). Temperature must be monitored closely because of the slight but described (LOE 2)[4] risk of hyperthermia with this technique. Other techniques to maintain temperature during stabilization of the infant in the delivery room (eg, drying and swaddling, warming pads, increased environmental temperature, placing the infant skin-to-skin with the mother and covering both with a blanket) have been used (LOE 8),[8,9] but they have not been evaluated in controlled trials nor compared with the plastic-wrap technique for premature infants. All resuscitation procedures, including endotracheal intubation, chest compression, and insertion of lines, can be performed with these temperature-controlling interventions in place.

Infants born to febrile mothers have been reported (LOE 4)[10–12] to have a higher incidence of perinatal respiratory depression, neonatal seizures, and cerebral palsy and increased risk of mortality. Animal studies (LOE 6)[13,14] indicate that hyperthermia during or after ischemia is associated with progression of cerebral injury. Hyperthermia should be avoided (Class IIb). The goal is to achieve normothermia and avoid iatrogenic hyperthermia.

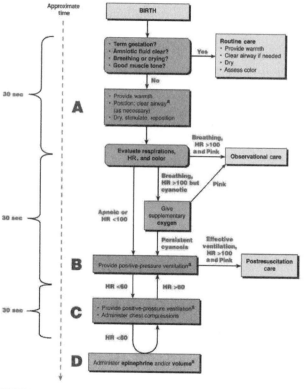

FIGURE 1

Neonatal flow algorithm. HR indicates heart rate (shown in bpm). [a] Endotracheal intubation may be considered at several steps.

CLEARING THE AIRWAY OF MECONIUM

Aspiration of meconium before delivery, during birth, or during resuscitation can cause severe aspiration pneumonia. One obstetrical technique to try to decrease aspiration has been to suction meconium from the infant's airway after delivery of the head but before delivery of the shoulders (intrapartum suctioning). Although some studies (LOE 3)[15–17] suggested that intrapartum suctioning might be effective for decreasing the risk of aspiration syndrome, subsequent evidence from a large multicenter randomized trial (LOE 1)[18] did not show such an effect. Therefore, current recommendations no longer advise routine intrapartum oropharyngeal and nasopharyngeal suctioning for infants born to mothers with meconium staining of amniotic fluid (Class I).

Traditional teaching (LOE 5)[19–21] recommended that meconium-stained infants have endotracheal intubation immediately following birth and that suction be applied to the endotracheal tube as it is withdrawn. Randomized, controlled trials (LOE 1)[15,22] have shown that this practice offers no benefit if the infant is vigorous (Class I). A vigorous infant is defined as one who has strong respiratory efforts, good muscle tone, and a heart rate >100 beats per minute (bpm). Endotracheal suctioning for infants who are not vigorous should be performed immediately after birth (Class Indeterminate).

PERIODIC EVALUATION AT 30-SECOND INTERVALS

After the immediate postbirth assessment and administration of initial steps, further resuscitative efforts should be guided by simultaneous assessment of respirations, heart rate, and color. After initial respiratory efforts the newly born infant should be able to establish regular respirations that are sufficient to improve color and maintain a heart rate >100 bpm. Gasping and apnea indicate the need for assisted ventilation.[23] Increasing or decreasing heart rate can also provide evidence of improvement or deterioration.

A newly born infant who is uncompromised will achieve and maintain pink mucous membranes without administration of supplementary oxygen. Evidence obtained with continuous oximetry, however, has shown that neonatal transition is a gradual process. Healthy infants born at term may take >10 minutes to achieve a preductal oxygen saturation >95% and nearly 1 hour to achieve postductal saturation >95% (LOE 5).[24–26] Central cyanosis is determined by examining the face, trunk, and mucous membranes. Acrocyanosis (blue color of hands and feet alone) is usually a normal finding at birth and is not a reliable indicator of hypoxemia but may indicate other conditions, such as cold stress. Pallor or mottling may be a sign of decreased cardiac output, severe anemia, hypovolemia, hypothermia, or acidosis.

ADMINISTRATION OF OXYGEN

There are concerns about the potential adverse effects of 100% oxygen on respiratory physiology and cerebral circulation and the potential tissue damage from oxygen free radicals. Conversely there are also concerns about tissue damage from oxygen deprivation during and after asphyxia. Studies (LOE 6)[27–31] examining blood pressure, cerebral perfusion, and various biochemical measures of cell damage in asphyxiated animals resuscitated with 100% oxygen versus 21% oxygen (room air) have shown conflicting results. One (LOE 2)[32] study of preterm infants (<33 weeks of gestation) exposed to 80% oxygen found lower cerebral blood flow when compared with those stabilized using 21% oxygen. Some animal data (LOE 6)[27] indicated the opposite effect, that is, reduced blood pressure and cerebral perfusion with 21% oxygen (room air) versus 100% oxygen. Meta-analysis of 4 human studies (LOE 1)[33,34] showed a reduction in mortality rate and no evidence of harm in infants resuscitated with room air versus those resuscitated with 100% oxygen, although these results should be viewed with caution because of significant methodologic concerns.

Supplementary oxygen is recommended whenever positive-pressure ventilation is indicated for resuscitation; free-flow oxygen should be administered to infants who are breathing but have central cyanosis (Class Indeterminate). The standard approach to resuscitation is to use 100% oxygen. Some clinicians may begin resuscitation with an oxygen concentration of less than 100%, and some may start with no supplementary oxygen (ie, room air). There is evidence that employing either of these practices during resuscitation of neonates is reasonable. If the clinician begins resuscitation with room air, it is recommended that supplementary oxygen be available to use if there is no appreciable improvement within 90 seconds after birth. In situations where supplementary oxygen is not readily available, positive-pressure ventilation should be administered with room air (Class Indeterminate).

Administration of a variable concentration of oxygen guided by pulse oximetry may improve the ability to achieve normoxia more quickly. Concerns about potential oxidant injury should caution the clinician about the use of excessive oxygen, especially in the premature infant.

POSITIVE-PRESSURE VENTILATION

If the infant remains apneic or gasping, if the heart rate remains <100 bpm 30 seconds after administering the initial steps, or if the infant continues to have persistent central cyanosis despite administration of supplementary oxygen, start positive-pressure ventilation.

INITIAL BREATHS AND ASSISTED VENTILATION

In term infants, initial inflations—either spontaneous or assisted—create a functional residual capacity (LOE 5).[35–41] The optimum pressure, inflation time, and flow rate required to establish an effective functional residual capacity have not been determined. Average initial peak inflating pressures of 30 to 40 cm H_2O (inflation time undefined) usually successfully ventilate unresponsive term infants (LOE 5).[36,38,40–43] Assisted ventilation rates of 40 to 60 breaths per minute are commonly used, but the relative efficacy of various rates has not been investigated.

The primary measure of adequate initial ventilation is prompt improvement in heart rate. Chest wall movement should be assessed if heart rate does not improve. The initial peak inflating pressures needed are variable and unpredictable and should be individualized to achieve an increase in heart rate and/or movement of the chest with each breath. If inflation pressure is being monitored, an initial inflation pressure of 20 cm H_2O may be effective, but $\geq$30 to 40 cm H_2O may be required in some term infants without spontaneous ventilation (Class IIb). If pressure is not monitored, the minimum inflation required to achieve an increase in heart rate should be used. There is insufficient evidence to recommend an optimum inflation time. In summary, assisted ventilation should be delivered at a rate of 40 to 60 breaths per minute (Class Indeterminate; LOE 8) to promptly achieve or maintain a heart rate >100 bpm.

DEVICES

Effective ventilation can be achieved with a flow-inflating bag, a self-inflating bag, or with a T-piece (LOE 4[44,45]; LOE 5[46]). A T-piece is a valved mechanical device designed to control flow and limit pressure. The pop-off valves of self-inflating bags are flow-dependent, and pressures generated may exceed the value specified by the manufacturer (LOE 6).[47] Target inflation pressures and long inspiratory times are more consistently achieved in mechanical models when T-piece devices are used rather than bags (LOE 6),[48] although the clinical implications are not clear. To provide the desired pressure, health care providers need more training in the use of flow-inflating bags than with self-inflating bags (LOE 6).[49] A self-inflating bag, a flow-inflating bag, or a T-piece can be used to ventilate a newborn (Class IIb).

Laryngeal mask airways (LMAs) that fit over the laryngeal inlet have been shown to be effective for ventilating newly born near-term and full-term infants (LOE 2[50] and LOE 5[51]). There are limited (LOE 5)[52,53] data on the use of these devices in small preterm infants. Data from 3 case series (LOE 5)[51,54,55] show that the use of the LMA can provide effective ventilation in a time frame consistent with current resuscitation guidelines, although the infants being studied were not being resuscitated. A randomized, controlled trial (LOE 2)[50] found no clinically significant difference between the use of the LMA and endotracheal intubation when bag-mask ventilation was unsuccessful. It is unclear whether this study can be generalized because the LMA was inserted by experienced providers. Case reports (LOE 5)[56–58] suggest that when bag-mask ventilation has been unsuccessful and endotracheal intubation is not feasible or is unsuccessful, the LMA may provide effective ventilation. There is insufficient evidence to support the routine use of the LMA as the primary airway device during neonatal resuscitation, in the setting of meconium-stained amniotic fluid, when chest compressions are required, in very low birth weight infants, or for delivery of emergency intratracheal medications (Class Indeterminate).

ASSISTED VENTILATION OF PRETERM INFANTS

Evidence from animal studies (LOE 6)[59] indicates that preterm lungs are easily injured by large-volume inflations immediately after birth. Additional animal studies (LOE 6)[60,61] indicate that when positive-pressure ventilation is applied immediately after birth, the inclusion of positive end-expiratory pressure protects against lung injury and improves lung compliance and gas exchange (LOE 6).[60,61] Evidence from case series in human infants indicates that most apneic preterm infants can be ventilated with an initial inflation pressure of 20 to 25 cm H_2O, although some infants who do not respond require a higher pressure (LOE 5).[62,63]

When ventilating preterm infants after birth, excessive chest wall movement may indicate large-volume lung inflations, which should be avoided. Monitoring of pressure may help to provide consistent inflations and avoid unnecessary high pressures (Class IIb). If positive-pressure ventilation is required, an initial inflation pressure of 20 to 25 cm H_2O is adequate for most preterm infants (Class Indeterminate). If prompt improvement in heart rate or chest movement is not obtained, higher pressures may be needed. If it is necessary to continue positive-pressure ventilation, application of positive end-expiratory pressure may be beneficial (Class Indeterminate). Continuous positive airway pressure in spontaneously breathing preterm infants after resuscitation may also be beneficial[63] (Class Indeterminate).

ENDOTRACHEAL TUBE PLACEMENT

Endotracheal intubation may be indicated at several points during neonatal resuscitation:

- When tracheal suctioning for meconium is required
- If bag-mask ventilation is ineffective or prolonged
- When chest compressions are performed
- When endotracheal administration of medications is desired

- For special resuscitation circumstances, such as congenital diaphragmatic hernia or extremely low birth weight (<1000 g)

The timing of endotracheal intubation may also depend on the skill and experience of the available providers.

After endotracheal intubation and administration of intermittent positive pressure, a prompt increase in heart rate is the best indicator that the tube is in the tracheobronchial tree and providing effective ventilation (LOE 5).[64] Exhaled CO_2 detection is effective for confirmation of endotracheal tube placement in infants, including very low birth weight infants (LOE 5).[65–68] A positive test result (detection of exhaled CO_2) in patients with adequate cardiac output confirms placement of the endotracheal tube within the trachea, whereas a negative test result (ie, no CO_2 detected) strongly suggests esophageal intubation (LOE 5).[65,67] Poor or absent pulmonary blood flow may give false-negative results (ie, no CO_2 detected despite tube placement in the trachea), but endotracheal tube placement is correctly identified in nearly all patients who are not in cardiac arrest (LOE 7).[69] A false-negative result may also lead to unnecessary extubation in critically ill infants with poor cardiac output.

Other clinical indicators of correct endotracheal tube placement are evaluation of condensed humidified gas during exhalation and the presence or absence of chest movement, but these have not been systematically evaluated in neonates. Endotracheal tube placement must be assessed visually during intubation and by confirmatory methods after intubation if the heart rate remains low and is not rising. Except for intubation to remove meconium, exhaled CO_2 detection is the recommended method of confirmation (Class IIa).

CHEST COMPRESSIONS

Chest compressions are indicated for a heart rate that is <60 bpm despite adequate ventilation with supplementary oxygen for 30 seconds. Because ventilation is the most effective action in neonatal resuscitation and because chest compressions are likely to compete with effective ventilation, rescuers should ensure that assisted ventilation is being delivered optimally before starting chest compressions.

Compressions should be delivered on the lower third of the sternum[70,71] to a depth of approximately one third of the anterior-posterior diameter of the chest. Two techniques have been described: compression with 2 thumbs with fingers encircling the chest and supporting the back[72–74] (the 2 thumb-encircling hands technique) or compression with 2 fingers with a second hand supporting the back. Because the 2 thumb-encircling hands technique may generate higher peak systolic and coronary perfusion pressure than the 2-finger technique

(LOE 5[75]; LOE 6[76]), the 2 thumb-encircling hands technique is recommended for performing chest compressions in newly born infants. However, the 2-finger technique may be preferable when access to the umbilicus is required during insertion of an umbilical catheter.

A compression/relaxation ratio with a slightly shorter compression than relaxation phase offers theoretical advantages for blood flow in the very young infant.[77] Also, compressions and ventilations should be coordinated to avoid simultaneous delivery (LOE 6).[78] The chest should be permitted to fully reexpand during relaxation, but the rescuer's thumbs should not leave the chest. There should be a 3:1 ratio of compressions to ventilations with 90 compressions and 30 breaths to achieve ~120 events per minute to maximize ventilation at an achievable rate (Class Indeterminate). Thus, each event will be allotted approximately ½ second, with exhalation occurring during the first compression after each ventilation.

Respirations, heart rate, and color should be reassessed about every 30 seconds, and coordinated chest compressions and ventilations should continue until the spontaneous heart rate is ≥60 bpm (Class IIa; LOE 8).

MEDICATIONS

Drugs are rarely indicated in resuscitation of the newly born infant.[79] Bradycardia in the newborn infant is usually the result of inadequate lung inflation or profound hypoxemia, and establishing adequate ventilation is the most important step to correct it. But if the heart rate remains <60 bpm despite adequate ventilation with 100% oxygen and chest compressions, administration of epinephrine or volume expansion, or both, may be indicated. Rarely, buffers, a narcotic antagonist, or vasopressors may be useful after resuscitation.

ROUTE AND DOSE OF EPINEPHRINE ADMINISTRATION

Past guidelines recommended that initial doses of epinephrine be given through an endotracheal tube because the dose can be administered more quickly than when an intravenous (IV) route must be established. However, animal studies (LOE 6)[80–82] that showed a positive effect of endotracheal epinephrine used considerably higher doses than are currently recommended, and the 1 animal study (LOE 6)[83] that used currently recommended doses given endotracheally showed no effect. Given the lack of data on endotracheal epinephrine, the IV route should be used as soon as venous access is established.

The recommended IV dose is 0.01 to 0.03 mg/kg per dose. Higher IV doses are not recommended (Class III) because animal (LOE 6)[84,85] and pediatric (LOE 7)[86] studies show exaggerated hypertension, decreased myocardial function, and worse neurologic function after administration of IV doses in the range of 0.1 mg/kg. If the endotracheal route is used, doses of 0.01 or 0.03 mg/kg will likely be ineffective. Therefore, IV administration of

0.01 to 0.03 mg/kg per dose is the preferred route (Class IIa). While access is being obtained, administration of a higher dose (up to 0.1 mg/kg) through the endotracheal tube may be considered (Class Indeterminate), but the safety and efficacy of this practice have not been evaluated. The concentration of epinephrine for either route should be 1:10 000 (0.1 mg/mL).

VOLUME EXPANSION

Consider volume expansion when blood loss is suspected or the infant appears to be in shock (pale skin, poor perfusion, weak pulse) and has not responded adequately to other resuscitative measures. An isotonic crystalloid rather than albumin is the solution of choice for volume expansion in the delivery room (Class IIb; LOE 7).[87–89] The recommended dose is 10 mL/kg, which may need to be repeated. When resuscitating premature infants, care should be taken to avoid giving volume expanders too rapidly, because rapid infusions of large volumes have been associated with intraventricular hemorrhage.

NALOXONE

Administration of naloxone is not recommended as part of initial resuscitative efforts in the delivery room for newborns with respiratory depression. If administration of naloxone is considered, heart rate and color must first be restored by supporting ventilation. The preferred route is IV or intramuscular. Given the lack of clinical data in newborns, endotracheal administration of naloxone is not recommended (Class Indeterminate). The recommended dose is 0.1 mg/kg, but no studies have examined the efficacy of this dose in newborns. In 1 case report, naloxone given to an infant born to an opioid-addicted mother was associated with seizures (LOE 8).[90] Therefore, naloxone should be avoided in infants whose mothers are suspected of having had long-term exposure to opioids (Class Indeterminate). Naloxone may have a shorter half-life than the original maternal opioid; therefore the neonate should be monitored closely for recurrent apnea or hypoventilation, and subsequent doses of naloxone may be required.

POSTRESUSCITATION CARE

Infants who require resuscitation are at risk for deterioration after their vital signs have returned to normal. Once adequate ventilation and circulation have been established, the infant should be maintained in or transferred to an environment in which close monitoring and anticipatory care can be provided.

GLUCOSE

Low blood glucose has been associated with adverse neurologic outcome in a neonatal animal model of asphyxia and resuscitation (LOE 6).[91] Neonatal animals (LOE 6)[92,93] that were hypoglycemic at the time of an anoxic or hypoxic-ischemic insult had larger areas of cerebral infarction or decreased survival, or both, when compared with controls. One clinical study (LOE 4)[94] showed an association between hypoglycemia and poor neurologic outcome after perinatal asphyxia.

No clinical neonatal studies have investigated the relation between hyperglycemia and neurologic outcome, although hyperglycemia in adults (LOE 7 [extrapolated][95]) is associated with worse outcome. The range of blood glucose concentration associated with the least brain injury after asphyxia and resuscitation cannot be defined based on available evidence. Infants who require significant resuscitation should be monitored and treated to maintain glucose in the normal range (Class Indeterminate).

INDUCED HYPOTHERMIA

In a multicenter trial (LOE 2)[96] involving newborns with suspected asphyxia (indicated by need for resuscitation at birth, metabolic acidosis, and early encephalopathy), selective head cooling (34–35°C) was associated with a nonsignificant reduction in the overall number of survivors with severe disability at 18 months but a significant benefit in the subgroup with moderate encephalopathy. Infants with severe electrographic suppression and seizures did not benefit from treatment with modest hypothermia (LOE 2).[96] A second large multicenter trial (LOE 2)[97] of asphyxiated newborns (indicated by need for resuscitation at birth or presence of metabolic encephalopathy) involved treatment with systemic hypothermia to 33.5°C (92.3°F) following moderate to severe encephalopathy. Hypothermia was associated with a significant (18%) decrease in death or moderate disability at 18 months.[97] A third small controlled pilot study (LOE 2)[98,99] in asphyxiated infants with early induced systemic hypothermia found fewer deaths and disability at 12 months.

Modest hypothermia is associated with bradycardia and elevated blood pressure that do not usually require treatment, but a rapid increase in body temperature may cause hypotension (LOE 5).[100] Cooling to a core temperature <33°C may cause arrhythmia, bleeding, thrombosis, and sepsis, but studies so far have not reported these complications in infants treated with modest (eg, 33–34.5°C [91.4–94.1°F]) hypothermia (LOE 2).[96,101]

There is insufficient data to recommend routine use of modest systemic or selective cerebral hypothermia after resuscitation of infants with suspected asphyxia (Class Indeterminate). Further clinical trials are needed to determine which infants benefit most and which method of cooling is most effective. Avoidance of hyperthermia (elevated body temperature) is particularly important in infants who may have had a hypoxic-ischemic event.

GUIDELINES FOR WITHHOLDING AND DISCONTINUING RESUSCITATION

Morbidity and mortality for newborns vary according to region and availability of resources (LOE 5).[102] Social science studies[103] indicate that parents desire a larger role in decisions to initiate resuscitation and continue life support of severely compromised newborns. Opinions among neonatal providers vary widely regarding the benefits and disadvantages of aggressive therapies in such newborns (LOE 5).[104]

WITHHOLDING RESUSCITATION

It is possible to identify conditions associated with high mortality and poor outcome in which withholding resuscitative efforts may be considered reasonable, particularly when there has been the opportunity for parental agreement (LOE 5).[2,105]

A consistent and coordinated approach to individual cases by the obstetric and neonatal teams and the parents is an important goal. Noninitiation of resuscitation and discontinuation of life-sustaining treatment during or after resuscitation are ethically equivalent, and clinicians should not hesitate to withdraw support when functional survival is highly unlikely. The following guidelines must be interpreted according to current regional outcomes:

- When gestation, birth weight, or congenital anomalies are associated with almost certain early death and when unacceptably high morbidity is likely among the rare survivors, resuscitation is not indicated (Class IIa). Examples may include extreme prematurity (gestational age <23 weeks or birth weight <400 g), anencephaly, and chromosomal abnormalities incompatible with life, such as trisomy 13.

- In conditions associated with a high rate of survival and acceptable morbidity, resuscitation is nearly always indicated (Class IIa). This will generally include infants with gestational age ≥25 weeks (unless there is evidence of fetal compromise such as intrauterine infection or hypoxia-ischemia) and those with most congenital malformations.

- In conditions associated with uncertain prognosis in which survival is borderline, the morbidity rate is relatively high, and the anticipated burden to the child is high, parental desires concerning initiation of resuscitation should be supported (Class Indeterminate).

DISCONTINUING RESUSCITATIVE EFFORTS

Infants without signs of life (no heart beat and no respiratory effort) after 10 minutes of resuscitation show either a high mortality or severe neurodevelopmental disability (LOE 5).[106,107] After 10 minutes of continuous and adequate resuscitative efforts, discontinuation of resuscitation may be justified if there are no signs of life (Class IIb).

NEONATAL RESUSCITATION GUIDELINES CONTRIBUTORS

John Kattwinkel, MD
Jeffrey M. Perlman, MB, ChB
David Boyle, MD
William A. Engle, MD
Marilyn Escobedo, MD
Jay P. Goldsmith, MD
Louis P. Halamek, MD
Jane McGowan, MD
Nalini Singhal, MD
Gary M. Weiner, MD
Thomas Wiswell, MD
Jeanette Zaichkin, RNC, MN
Wendy Marie Simon, MA, CAE

ACKNOWLEDGMENTS

The American Academy of Pediatrics Neonatal Resuscitation Program Steering Committee would like to acknowledge the seminal contribution of John Kattwinkel, MD, to this document.

REFERENCES

1. American Academy of Pediatrics, American College of Obstetricians and Gynecologists. In: Gilstrap LC, Oh W, eds. *Guidelines for Perinatal Care*. 5th ed. Elk Grove Village, IL: American Academy of Pediatrics; 2002:187
2. Costeloe K, Hennessy E, Gibson AT, Marlow N, Wilkinson AR. The EPICure study: outcomes to discharge from hospital for infants born at the threshold of viability. *Pediatrics*. 2000;106:659–671
3. Vohra S, Frent G, Campbell V, Abbott M, Whyte R. Effect of polyethylene occlusive skin wrapping on heat loss in very low birth weight infants at delivery: a randomized trial. *J Pediatr*. 1999;134:547–551
4. Vohra S, Roberts RS, Zhang B, Janes M, Schmidt B. Heat Loss Prevention (HeLP) in the delivery room: a randomized controlled trial of polyethylene occlusive skin wrapping in very preterm infants. *J Pediatr*. 2004;145:750–753
5. Lyon AJ, Stenson B. Cold comfort for babies. *Arch Dis Child Fetal Neonatal Ed*. 2004;89:F93–F94
6. Lenclen R, Mazraani M, Jugie M, et al. Use of a polyethylene bag: a way to improve the thermal environment of the premature newborn at the delivery room [in French]. *Arch Pediatr*. 2002;9:238–244
7. Bjorklund LJ, Hellstrom-Westas L. Reducing heat loss at birth in very preterm infants. *J Pediatr*. 2000;137:739–740
8. Baum JD, Scopes JW. The silver swaddler: device for preventing hypothermia in the newborn. *Lancet*. 1968;1(7544):672–673
9. Besch NJ, Perlstein PH, Edwards NK, Keenan WJ, Sutherland JM. The transparent baby bag: a shield against heat loss. *N Engl J Med*. 1971;284:121–124
10. Petrova A, Demissie K, Rhoads GG, Smulian JC, Marcella S, Ananth CV. Association of maternal fever during labor with neonatal and infant morbidity and mortality. *Obstet Gynecol*. 2001;98:20–27
11. Lieberman E, Lang J, Richardson DK, Frigoletto FD, Heffner LJ, Cohen A. Intrapartum maternal fever and neonatal outcome. *Pediatrics*. 2000;105:8–13

12. Grether JK, Nelson KB. Maternal infection and cerebral palsy in infants of normal birth weight. *JAMA.* 1997;278:207–211

13. Coimbra C, Boris-Moller F, Drake M, Wieloch T. Diminished neuronal damage in the rat brain by late treatment with the antipyretic drug dipyrone or cooling following cerebral ischemia. *Acta Neuropathol (Berl).* 1996;92:447–453

14. Dietrich WD, Alonso O, Halley M, Busto R. Delayed posttraumatic brain hyperthermia worsens outcome after fluid percussion brain injury: a light and electron microscopic study in rats. *Neurosurgery.* 1996;38:533–541; discussion 541

15. Wiswell TE, Gannon CM, Jacob J, et al. Delivery room management of the apparently vigorous meconium-stained neonate: results of the multicenter, international collaborative trial. *Pediatrics.* 2000;105:1–7

16. Falciglia HS, Henderschott C, Potter P, Helmchen R. Does DeLee suction at the perineum prevent meconium aspiration syndrome? *Am J Obstet Gynecol.* 1992;167:1243–1249

17. Carson BS, Losey RW, Bowes WA Jr, Simmons MA. Combined obstetric and pediatric approach to prevent meconium aspiration syndrome. *Am J Obstet Gynecol.* 1976;126:712–715

18. Vain NE, Szyld EG, Prudent LM, Wiswell TE, Aguilar AM, Vivas NI. Oropharyngeal and nasopharyngeal suctioning of meconium-stained neonates before delivery of their shoulders: multicentre, randomised controlled trial. *Lancet.* 2004;364:597–602

19. Gregory GA, Gooding CA, Phibbs RH, Tooley WH. Meconium aspiration in infants: a prospective study. *J Pediatr.* 1974;85:848–852

20. Rossi EM, Philipson EH, Williams TG, Kalhan SC. Meconium aspiration syndrome: intrapartum and neonatal attributes. *Am J Obstet Gynecol.* 1989;161:1106–1110

21. Davis RO, Philips JB III, Harris BA Jr, Wilson ER, Huddleston JF. Fatal meconium aspiration syndrome occurring despite airway management considered appropriate. *Am J Obstet Gynecol.* 1985;151:731–736

22. Halliday HL. Endotracheal intubation at birth for preventing morbidity and mortality in vigorous, meconium-stained infants born at term. *Cochrane Database Syst Rev.* 2001;(1):CD000500

23. Dawes GS. *Foetal and Neonatal Physiology: A Comparative Study of the Changes at Birth.* Chicago, IL: Year Book Medical Publishers Inc; 1968

24. Harris AP, Sendak MJ, Donham RT. Changes in arterial oxygen saturation immediately after birth in the human neonate. *J Pediatr.* 1986;109:117–119

25. Reddy VK, Holzman IR, Wedgwood JF. Pulse oximetry saturations in the first 6 hours of life in normal term infants. *Clin Pediatr (Phila).* 1999;38:87–92

26. Toth B, Becker A, Seelbach-Gobel B. Oxygen saturation in healthy newborn infants immediately after birth measured by pulse oximetry. *Arch Gynecol Obstet.* 2002;266:105–107

27. Solas AB, Kutzsche S, Vinje M, Saugstad OD. Cerebral hypoxemia-ischemia and reoxygenation with 21% or 100% oxygen in newborn piglets: effects on extracellular levels of excitatory amino acids and microcirculation. *Pediatr Crit Care Med.* 2001;2:340–345

28. Solas AB, Munkeby BH, Saugstad OD. Comparison of short- and long-duration oxygen treatment after cerebral asphyxia in newborn piglets. *Pediatr Res.* 2004;56:125–131

29. Solas AB, Kalous P, Saugstad OD. Reoxygenation with 100 or 21% oxygen after cerebral hypoxemia-ischemia-hypercapnia in newborn piglets. *Biol Neonate.* 2004;85:105–111

30. Huang CC, Yonetani M, Lajevardi N, Delivoria-Papadopoulos M, Wilson DF, Pastuszko A. Comparison of postasphyxial resuscitation with 100% and 21% oxygen on cortical oxygen pressure and striatal dopamine metabolism in newborn piglets. *J Neurochem.* 1995;64:292–298

31. Kutzsche S, Kirkeby OJ, Rise IR, Saugstad OD. Effects of hypoxia and reoxygenation with 21% and 100%-oxygen on cerebral nitric oxide concentration and microcirculation in newborn piglets. *Biol Neonate.* 1999;76:153–167

32. Lundstrom KE, Pryds O, Greisen G. Oxygen at birth and prolonged cerebral vasoconstriction in preterm infants. *Arch Dis Child Fetal Neonatal Ed.* 1995;73:F81–F86

33. Tan A, Schulze A, O'Donnell CP, Davis PG. Air versus oxygen for resuscitation of infants at birth. *Cochrane Database Syst Rev.* 2005;(2):CD002273

34. Davis PG, Tan A, O'Donnell CP, Schulze A. Resuscitation of newborn infants with 100% oxygen or air: a systematic review and meta-analysis. *Lancet.* 2004;364:1329–1333

35. Karlberg P, Koch G. Respiratory studies in newborn infants, III: development of mechanics of breathing during the first week of life. A longitudinal study. *Acta Paediatr.* 1962;(suppl 135):121–129

36. Vyas H, Milner AD, Hopkin IE, Boon AW. Physiologic responses to prolonged and slow-rise inflation in the resuscitation of the asphyxiated newborn infant. *J Pediatr.* 1981;99:635–639

37. Vyas H, Field D, Milner AD, Hopkin IE. Determinants of the first inspiratory volume and functional residual capacity at birth. *Pediatr Pulmonol.* 1986;2:189–193

38. Boon AW, Milner AD, Hopkin IE. Lung expansion, tidal exchange, and formation of the functional residual capacity during resuscitation of asphyxiated neonates. *J Pediatr.* 1979;95:1031–1036

39. Mortola JP, Fisher JT, Smith JB, Fox GS, Weeks S, Willis D. Onset of respiration in infants delivered by cesarean section. *J Appl Physiol.* 1982;52:716–724

40. Hull D. Lung expansion and ventilation during resuscitation of asphyxiated newborn infants. *J Pediatr.* 1969;75:47–58

41. Upton CJ, Milner AD. Endotracheal resuscitation of neonates using a rebreathing bag. *Arch Dis Child.* 1991;66:39–42

42. Boon AW, Milner AD, Hopkin IE. Physiological responses of the newborn infant to resuscitation. *Arch Dis Child.* 1979;54:492–498

43. Milner AD, Vyas H, Hopkin IE. Efficacy of facemask resuscitation at birth. *BMJ.* 1984;289:1563–1565

44. Allwood AC, Madar RJ, Baumer JH, Readdy L, Wright D. Changes in resuscitation practice at birth. *Arch Dis Child Fetal Neonatal Ed.* 2003;88:F375–F379

45. Hoskyns EW, Milner AD, Hopkin IE. A simple method of face mask resuscitation at birth. *Arch Dis Child.* 1987;62:376–378

46. Cole AF, Rolbin SH, Hew EM, Pynn S. An improved ventilator system for delivery-room management of the newborn. *Anesthesiology.* 1979;51:356–358

47. Ganga-Zandzou PS, Diependaele JF, Storme L, et al. Is Ambu ventilation of newborn infants a simple question of finger-touch [in French]? *Arch Pediatr.* 1996;3:1270–1272

48. Finer NN, Rich W, Craft A, Henderson C. Comparison of methods of bag and mask ventilation for neonatal resuscitation. *Resuscitation.* 2001;49:299–305

49. Kanter RK. Evaluation of mask-bag ventilation in resuscitation of infants. *Am J Dis Child.* 1987;141:761–763

50. Esmail N, Saleh M, Ali A. Laryngeal mask airway versus endotracheal intubation for Apgar score improvement in neonatal resuscitation. *Egyptian J Anesthesiol.* 2002;18:115–121

51. Gandini D, Brimacombe JR. Neonatal resuscitation with the laryngeal mask airway in normal and low birth weight infants. *Anesth Analg.* 1999;89:642–643

52. Brimacombe J, Gandini D. Airway rescue and drug delivery in an 800 g neonate with the laryngeal mask airway. *Paediatr Anaesth.* 1999;9:178

53. Lonnqvist PA. Successful use of laryngeal mask airway in low-weight expremature infants with bronchopulmonary

dysplasia undergoing cryotherapy for retinopathy of the premature. *Anesthesiology.* 1995;83:422–424

54. Paterson SJ, Byrne PJ, Molesky MG, Seal RF, Finucane BT. Neonatal resuscitation using the laryngeal mask airway. *Anesthesiology.* 1994;80:1248–1253

55. Trevisanuto D, Ferrarese P, Zanardo V, Chiandetti L. Laryngeal mask airway in neonatal resuscitation: a survey of current practice and perceived role by anaesthesiologists and paediatricians. *Resuscitation.* 2004;60:291–296

56. Hansen TG, Joensen H, Henneberg SW, Hole P. Laryngeal mask airway guided tracheal intubation in a neonate with the Pierre Robin syndrome. *Acta Anaesthesiol Scand.* 1995;39: 129–131

57. Osses H, Poblete M, Asenjo F. Laryngeal mask for difficult intubation in children. *Paediatr Anaesth.* 1999;9:399–401

58. Stocks RM, Egerman R, Thompson JW, Peery M. Airway management of the severely retrognathic child: use of the laryngeal mask airway. *Ear Nose Throat J.* 2002;81:223–226

59. Ingimarsson J, Bjorklund LJ, Curstedt T, et al. Incomplete protection by prophylactic surfactant against the adverse effects of large lung inflations at birth in immature lambs. *Intensive Care Med.* 2004;30:1446–1453

60. Nilsson R, Grossmann G, Robertson B. Bronchiolar epithelial lesions induced in the premature rabbit neonate by short periods of artificial ventilation. *Acta Pathol Microbiol Scand [A].* 1980;88:359–367

61. Probyn ME, Hooper SB, Dargaville PA, et al. Positive end expiratory pressure during resuscitation of premature lambs rapidly improves blood gases without adversely affecting arterial pressure. *Pediatr Res.* 2004;56:198–204

62. Hird MF, Greenough A, Gamsu HR. Inflating pressures for effective resuscitation of preterm infants. *Early Hum Dev.* 1991;26:69–72

63. Lindner W, Vossbeck S, Hummler H, Pohlandt F. Delivery room management of extremely low birth weight infants: spontaneous breathing or intubation? *Pediatrics.* 1999;103: 961–967

64. Palme-Kilander C, Tunell R. Pulmonary gas exchange during facemask ventilation immediately after birth. *Arch Dis Child.* 1993;68:11–16

65. Aziz HF, Martin JB, Moore JJ. The pediatric disposable end-tidal carbon dioxide detector role in endotracheal intubation in newborns. *J Perinatol.* 1999;19:110–113

66. Bhende MS, Thompson AE. Evaluation of an end-tidal CO2 detector during pediatric cardiopulmonary resuscitation. *Pediatrics.* 1995;95:395–399

67. Repetto JE, Donohue PCP, Baker SF, Kelly L, Nogee LM. Use of capnography in the delivery room for assessment of endotracheal tube placement. *J Perinatol.* 2001;21:284–287

68. Roberts WA, Maniscalco WM, Cohen AR, Litman RS, Chhibber A. The use of capnography for recognition of esophageal intubation in the neonatal intensive care unit. *Pediatr Pulmonol.* 1995;19:262–268

69. Bhende MS, Karasic DG, Karasic RB. End-tidal carbon dioxide changes during cardiopulmonary resuscitation after experimental asphyxial cardiac arrest. *Am J Emerg Med.* 1996;14: 349–350

70. Orlowski JP. Optimum position for external cardiac compression in infants and young children. *Ann Emerg Med.* 1986;15: 667–673

71. Phillips GW, Zideman DA. Relation of infant heart to sternum: its significance in cardiopulmonary resuscitation. *Lancet.* 1986;1(8488):1024–1025

72. Thaler MM, Stobie GH. An improved technique of external cardiac compression in infants and young children. *N Engl J Med.* 1963;269:606–610

73. David R. Closed chest cardiac massage in the newborn infant. *Pediatrics.* 1988;81:552–554

74. Todres ID, Rogers MC. Methods of external cardiac massage in the newborn infant. *J Pediatr.* 1975;86:781–782

75. Menegazzi JJ, Auble TE, Nicklas KA, Hosack GM, Rack L, Goode JS. Two-thumb versus two-finger chest compression during CRP in a swine infant model of cardiac arrest. *Ann Emerg Med.* 1993;22:240–243

76. Houri PK, Frank LR, Menegazzi JJ, Taylor R. A randomized, controlled trial of two-thumb vs two-finger chest compression in a swine infant model of cardiac arrest. *Prehosp Emerg Care.* 1997;1:65–67

77. Dean JM, Koehler RC, Schleien CL, et al. Age-related effects of compression rate and duration in cardiopulmonary resuscitation. *J Appl Physiol.* 1990;68:554–560

78. Berkowitz ID, Chantarojanasiri T, Koehler RC, et al. Blood flow during cardiopulmonary resuscitation with simultaneous compression and ventilation in infant pigs. *Pediatr Res.* 1989;26:558–564

79. Perlman JM, Risser R. Cardiopulmonary resuscitation in the delivery room: associated clinical events. *Arch Pediatr Adolesc Med.* 1995;149:20–25

80. Ralston SH, Voorhees WD, Babbs CF. Intrapulmonary epinephrine during prolonged cardiopulmonary resuscitation: improved regional blood flow and resuscitation in dogs. *Ann Emerg Med.* 1984;13:79–86

81. Ralston SH, Tacker WA, Showen L, Carter A, Babbs CF. Endotracheal versus intravenous epinephrine during electromechanical dissociation with CPR in dogs. *Ann Emerg Med.* 1985;14:1044–1048

82. Redding JS, Pearson JW. Metabolic acidosis: a factor in cardiac resuscitation. *South Med J.* 1967;60:926–932

83. Kleinman ME, Oh W, Stonestreet BS. Comparison of intravenous and endotracheal epinephrine during cardiopulmonary resuscitation in newborn piglets. *Crit Care Med.* 1999;27: 2748–2754

84. Berg RA, Otto CW, Kern KB, et al. A randomized, blinded trial of high-dose epinephrine versus standard-dose epinephrine in a swine model of pediatric asphyxial cardiac arrest. *Crit Care Med.* 1996;24:1695–1700

85. Burchfield DJ, Preziosi MP, Lucas VW, Fan J. Effects of graded doses of epinephrine during asphyxia-induced bradycardia in newborn lambs. *Resuscitation.* 1993;25:235–244

86. Perondi MB, Reis AG, Paiva EF, Nadkarni VM, Berg RA. A comparison of high-dose and standard-dose epinephrine in children with cardiac arrest. *N Engl J Med.* 2004;350: 1722–1730

87. So KW, Fok TF, Ng PC, Wong WW, Cheung KL. Randomised controlled trial of colloid or crystalloid in hypotensive preterm infants. *Arch Dis Child Fetal Neonatal Ed.* 1997;76:F43–F46

88. Emery EF, Greenough A, Gamsu HR. Randomised controlled trial of colloid infusions in hypotensive preterm infants. *Arch Dis Child.* 1992;67:1185–1188

89. Oca MJ, Nelson M, Donn SM. Randomized trial of normal saline versus 5% albumin for the treatment of neonatal hypotension. *J Perinatol.* 2003;23:473–476

90. Gibbs J, Newson T, Williams J, Davidson DC. Naloxone hazard in infant of opioid abuser. *Lancet.* 1989;2(8655):159–160

91. Brambrink AM, Ichord RN, Martin LJ, Koehler RC, Traystman RJ. Poor outcome after hypoxia-ischemia in newborns is associated with physiological abnormalities during early recovery: possible relevance to secondary brain injury after head trauma in infants. *Exp Toxicol Pathol.* 1999;51:151–162

92. Vannucci RC, Vannucci SJ. Cerebral carbohydrate metabolism during hypoglycemia and anoxia in newborn rats. *Ann Neurol.* 1978;4:73–79

93. Yager JY, Heitjan DF, Towfighi J, Vannucci RC. Effect of insulin-induced and fasting hypoglycemia on perinatal hypoxic-ischemic brain damage. *Pediatr Res.* 1992;31:138–142

94. Salhab WA, Wyckoff MH, Laptook AR, Perlman JM. Initial hypoglycemia and neonatal brain injury in term infants with severe fetal acidemia. *Pediatrics.* 2004;114:361–366

95. Kent TA, Soukup VM, Fabian RH. Heterogeneity affecting outcome from acute stroke therapy: making reperfusion worse. *Stroke.* 2001;32:2318–2327

96. Gluckman PD, Wyatt JS, Azzopardi D, et al. Selective head cooling with mild systemic hypothermia after neonatal encephalopathy: multicentre randomised trial. *Lancet.* 2005; 365:663–670

97. Donovan EF, Fanaroff AA, Poole WK, et al. Whole-body hypothermia for neonates with hypoxic-ischemic encephalopathy. *N Engl J Med.* 2005;353:1574–1584

98. Eicher DJ, Wagner CL, Katikaneni LP, et al. Moderate hypothermia in neonatal encephalopathy: safety outcomes. *Pediatr Neurol.* 2005;32:18–24

99. Eicher DJ, Wagner CL, Katikaneni LP, et al. Moderate hypothermia in neonatal encephalopathy: efficacy outcomes. *Pediatr Neurol.* 2005;32:11–17

100. Thoresen M, Whitelaw A. Cardiovascular changes during mild therapeutic hypothermia and rewarming in infants with hypoxic-ischemic encephalopathy. *Pediatrics.* 2000;106:92–99

101. Shankaran S, Laptook A, Wright LL, et al. Whole-body hypothermia for neonatal encephalopathy: animal observations as a basis for a randomized, controlled pilot study in term infants. *Pediatrics.* 2002;110:377–385

102. De Leeuw R, Cuttini M, Nadai M, et al. Treatment choices for extremely preterm infants: an international perspective. *J Pediatr.* 2000;137:608–616

103. Lee SK, Penner PL, Cox M. Comparison of the attitudes of health care professionals and parents toward active treatment of very low birth weight infants. *Pediatrics.* 1991;88:110–114

104. Kopelman LM, Irons TG, Kopelman AE. Neonatologists judge the "Baby Doe" regulations. *N Engl J Med.* 1988;318:677–683

105. Draper ES, Manktelow B, Field DJ, James D. Tables for predicting survival for preterm births are updated. *BMJ.* 2003; 327:872

106. Jain L, Ferre C, Vidyasagar D, Nath S, Sheftel D. Cardiopulmonary resuscitation of apparently stillborn infants: survival and long-term outcome. *J Pediatr.* 1991;118:778–782

107. Haddad B, Mercer BM, Livingston JC, Talati A, Sibai BM. Outcome after successful resuscitation of babies born with Apgar scores of 0 at both 1 and 5 minutes. *Am J Obstet Gynecol.* 2000;182:1210–1214

Index

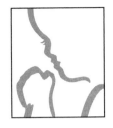

Index

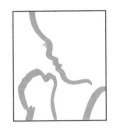

H

Hands, position of
 in 2-finger technique, 4-7
 on chest in beginning chest
  compressions, 4-5
 in thumb technique, 4-6–4-7
Heart disease, congenital, 6-12, 7-9
 cyanotic, 2-17
Heart murmurs, 7-14
Heart rate
 actions on abnormal, 2-14
 in evaluating newborn, 2-13
 stopping chest compressions and,
  4-12
Heat loss, preventing, 2-10
Hernia, congenital diaphragmatic, 7-3,
  7-6, 7-8
High-risk birth
 discussions with parents prior to, 9-7
 personnel needed at anticipated, 1-17
 prenatal counseling with parents
  prior to, 9-7–9-9
Hospital, neonatal resuscitation for
  babies born outside of, 7-18
Hyperoxic re-perfusion injury, 8-8
Hypertension, pulmonary, 7-13
Hyperthermia, 7-15
Hypocalcemia, 7-15
Hypoglycemia, 1-7, 7-15
Hypoplasia, pulmonary, 7-3, 7-9
Hypotension, 7-14, 7-15
 systemic, 1-6
Hypovolemia, 6-12
 acute, 6-10
 treating, 6-10
Hypovolemic shock, 6-10
Hypoxemia, 1-6, 2-13
Hypoxia, 1-6
 complication of, in endotracheal
  intubation, 5-25
Hypoxic-ischemic encephalopathy
  (HIE), 7-10, 7-14–7-15

I

Ileus, 7-15
Immaturity, extreme, 7-3, 7-9
Infection
 complication of, in endotracheal
  intubation, 5-25
 increased suspicion for, 8-12
Infectious agents, transmission of, 1-17
Inflation pressures, indication of
  adequate, 3-21
Inotropic agents, infusion of, 7-14
Inspiratory pressure
 control in T-piece resuscitator, 3-54
 inadequate, 3-24
Inspiratory time

capability to control, 3-10
 duration of, 3-10
Interosseous access as alternative to
  intravenous access for
  administration of medications,
  6-6
Intrapartum factors, need for neonatal
  resuscitation and, 1-15
Intravenous access, establishing, during
  newborn resuscitation, 6-4–6-5
Intubation equipment, 1-26
In utero compromise, 1-8–1-9
In vitro fertilization, 9-6
Ischemia, 1-6

L

Laryngeal mask airway
 defined, 5-38
 function of, 5-38
 indications of proper placement, 5-42
 inserting, 5-3, 5-40–5-41
 limitations of, 5-39
 possible complications with, 5-42
 preparing, 5-40
 reasons for using, 5-38–5-39
 removal of, 5-42
 securing and ventilating through, 5-42
 sizes of, 5-40
Laryngeal webs, 7-3, 7-5
Laryngoscope, in endotracheal
  intubation, 5-4
 hold of, 5-12
 preparing, 5-7–5-8
Larynx, 5-38
Life support, following neonatal
  resuscitation, 9-10
Lungs
 complications, 7-13
 failure of positive-pressure
  ventilation to result in
  adequate ventilation of, 7-3
 fetal, 1-4
 impaired functions of, 7-3, 7-6–7-9

M

Magnesium sulfate, 7-10
Main bronchi, 5-9
Malformation, congenital, 7-2, 7-5
Masks, sizes of, in positive-pressure
  ventilation, 3-10
Maximum pressure relief control in
  T-piece resuscitator, 3-54
Mechanical blockage of airway, 7-3,
  7-4–7-5
Meconium, 1-6
 blockage, 7-4
 need for endotracheal intubation
  and, 5-2

in pharynx or trachea, 7-3
 presence of
  in amniotic fluid, 2-4
  in nonvigorous baby, 2-6–2-7
  in vigorous baby, 2-7
 resuscitation involving, 2-3
 suctioning of, 5-15
  insertion of endotracheal tube
   and, 5-16
Meconium aspiration syndrome, 2-6
Meconium aspirator in endotracheal
  intubation, 5-4
Medications, 6-1–6-21
 adrenaline chloride, 6-6
 alternatives to intravenous access for
  administration of, during
  resuscitation of newborn, 6-6
 atropine, 6-4
 epinephrine, 5-2, 6-4, 6-5, 7-21
  administration of, 6-6–6-7
  amount to be given, 6-7
  on nonimprovement of newborn,
   4-13
  preparing, 6-7
  results on administration, 6-9
  via endotracheal tube,
   performance checklist and,
   6-21
 establishing intravenous access
  during resuscitation of
  newborn, 6-4–6-5
 expansion of blood volume, 6-10
 infusion of dopamine, 7-14
 lack of improvement, 6-12
 magnesium sulfate, 7-10
 naloxone, 6-4
 for neonatal resuscitation, 1-26
 nitric oxide, 7-13
 performance checklist and, 6-17
 resuscitation with positive-pressure
  ventilation, chest
  compressions, and, 6-2–6-3
 shock and, 6-10
 via umbilical vein, performance
  checklist and, 6-18–6-20
Metabolic acidosis, 7-13
Methadone maintenance, 7-10
Mortality, 9-2
Mouth
 anomalies of, and need for laryngeal
  mask airway, 5-38
 suctioning of, 2-9
Mucus blockage, 7-4
Mucus in pharynx or trachea, 7-3
Multiple births, personnel present at,
  1-16
Muscle tone, 1-14, 2-4
Myocardial function, deterioration
  of, 1-9

medications and, 6-17

medications via umbilical vein and, 6-18–6-20

for positive-pressure ventilation, 3-40–3-43

Perinatal compromise, 1-8–1-9, 1-18

Perinatal death, support for staff in nursing after, 9-12

Perinatal loss support group, 9-12

Peripheral vasoconstriction, 6-6

Persistent pulmonary hypertension of newborn, 1-7, 2-17

Pharyngeal airway malformation, 7-3, 7-4–7-5

Pharynx, anomalies of, and need for laryngeal mask airway, 5-38

Phenobarbital, 7-15

Placental abruption, 6-10

need for resuscitation with positive-pressure ventilation, chest compressions, medications and, 6-2–6-3

Placental membrane, 1-4

Placenta previa, 6-10

Plastic-bag technique, 8-6

Pleural effusions, 7-6–7-7

Pneumonia, 7-13

congenital, 7-3, 7-9

neonatal, 7-13

Pneumothorax, 6-12, 7-3, 7-6, 7-7, 7-13

complication of, in endotracheal intubation, 5-25

Pop-off valve, 3-8, 3-11

Positive end-expiratory pressure (PEEP), 3-5, 3-6, 3-7

assisting ventilation, 8-10–8-11

Positive end-expiratory pressure (PEEP) cap in T-piece resuscitator, 3-54

Positive-pressure device

in endotracheal intubation, 5-4

preparing, for administering, 5-8

Positive-pressure ventilation, 1-9, 1-17, 2-11, 3-2, 5-2, 7-19

advantages and disadvantages of assisted-ventilation devices, 3-7–3-8

characteristics of face masks in, 3-16

characteristics of resuscitation devices in, 3-10–3-11

checks before beginning, 3-18–3-19

concentration of oxygen used, 3-14

controls of respiratory limits during, with resuscitation devices, 3-12

failure in achieving adequate ventilation of lungs, 7-3

giving free-flow oxygen using resuscitation devices, 3-15

indications of improvement, 3-23–3-24

insertion of orogastric tube, 3-27–3-28

lack of improvement with, 3-29–3-30

medication and, 6-2–6-3

need for orogastric tube, 3-26–3-27

performance checklist, 3-40–3-43

preparing resuscitation devices for, 3-17

proper ventilation rate in, 3-22

resuscitation with chest compressions and, 4-2–4-3, 6-2–6-3

safety features of resuscitation devices, 3-11–3-12

signs of effective, 3-9

types of resuscitation devices for, 3-5–3-7

use of resuscitation devices for, 3-1–3-58

Post-resuscitation care, 7-12, 7-16

following neonatal resuscitation, 1-18

Premature babies

risk factors for, 1-16

vulnerability of, to injury from excess oxygen, 2-17

Premature newborn, length of trachea in, 5-5

Pressure, controlling in self-inflating bag, 3-47

Pressure-gauge attachment site in flow-inflating resuscitation bags, 3-48

Pressure gauge in self-inflating resuscitation bags, 3-44

Pressure-release valve, 3-8

in self-inflating resuscitation bags, 3-44

Preterm babies

evaluation of, 2-4

lungs of, 2-4

Primary apnea, 1-8, 2-11

Prophylactic administration of surfactant, 8-11

Pulmonary arterioles, sustained constriction of, 1-7

Pulmonary hypertension, 7-13

Pulmonary hypoplasia, 7-3, 7-9

Pulse oximeter, 7-19, 8-5, 8-9

R

Radiant warmer, 3-2

Reflex irritability, 1-14

Respirations

actions on abnormal, 2-14

in evaluating newborn, 2-13

failure to begin spontaneous, 7-10

Respiratory distress, 7-6

Resuscitation. *See also* Neonatal resuscitation

of apparently healthy newborn, 7-19

with bag and mask and oxygen, 3-2–3-3

complications after initial attempts at, 7-2

discontinuation of, 9-10

flow diagram, 1-10–1-12

initial steps in, 2-24–2-26

involving meconium, 2-3

maintaining body temperature during, 1-2

with positive-pressure ventilation, chest compressions and, 4-2–4-3

preparing for, 2-10

of preterm babies, 8-1–8-16

assisting ventilation, 8-10–8-11

decreasing chances of brain injury, 8-11–8-12

keeping baby warm, 8-6

oxygen use and, 8-8–8-9

reasons for high risk, 8-4

resources needed, 8-4–8-5

special precautions following, 8-12

stabilization of extremely preterm, 8-2–8-3

principles of, 1-1–1-28

steps in, 2-1–2-26

Resuscitation devices

characteristics of, 3-10–3-11

controls of respiratory limits during positive-pressure ventilation with, 3-12

preparing, for anticipated resuscitation, 3-17

safety features of, 3-11–3-12

use of, for positive-pressure ventilation, 3-1–3-58

Resuscitation team, 1-16

Robin syndrome, 7-3, 7-4–7-5, 7-5

need for laryngeal mask airway and, 5-38

Routine care, following neonatal resuscitation, 1-18

Textbook of Neonatal Resuscitation, 5th Edition
Evaluation

1. In which Neonatal Resuscitation Program (NRP) course did you use the *Textbook of Neonatal Resuscitation, 5th Edition?*
   ☐ Standard Provider Course ☐ Provider Renewal Course ☐ Instructor Course with a Provider Component

2. Please indicate your medical credentials.
   MD DO RN NNP RT PA EMT-P   EMT Other (please indicate): _____

3. Have you previously taken an NRP course?   ☐ Yes   ☐ No

4. Please use the scale below to rate the *Textbook of Neonatal Resuscitation, 5th Edition,* on the qualities listed.

   1 = Strongly Disagree   **2** = Disagree   **3** = Agree   **4** = Strongly Agree

	1	2	3	4
The textbook was well written.	1	2	3	4
The textbook effectively communicates the principles of the Neonatal Resuscitation Program.	1	2	3	4
The resuscitation flow diagram is easy to use.	1	2	3	4
Information follows a logical sequence from lesson to lesson.	1	2	3	4
The textbook adequately prepares a health care professional to participate in a neonatal resuscitation.	1	2	3	4
The case scenarios are useful.	1	2	3	4
The illustrations are useful.	1	2	3	4
The Performance Checklists match the course content.	1	2	3	4
The Megacode fosters skill integration.	1	2	3	4
The textbook is attractive and well designed.	1	2	3	4
The color photo section is useful.	1	2	3	4
The overall design of the textbook supports independent learning.	1	2	3	4
The practice activities aid in the learning process.	1	2	3	4

5. Have you used the *Textbook of Neonatal Resuscitation, 5th Edition, Multimedia DVD-ROM?* ☐ Yes ☐ No

   5a. If you answered no to the above question, do you plan to view the DVD-ROM?   ☐ Yes ☐ No

   5b. If you answered yes to the above question, feel free to include any comments about the DVD-ROM below.

   _____
   _____
   _____
   _____
   _____

6. What aspects or features of the textbook enhanced your learning?

   _____
   _____
   _____
   _____

7. How could the textbook be improved?

   _____
   _____
   _____
   _____

missed
picture of -
(1) vocal cords
glottis
epiglottis
valvulus

3 things to assess for skin color   is the baby term
                              HR
                        muscle tone

when not to resuscitate
          386 gm - don't have to resuscitate